Praise for *Shameless Sex*

"When it comes to talking about sex, Amy and April aren't just shameless—they're warm, wise, energetic, and empathetic. Now they've made the leap from podcast to page, and their new book is a dynamo of high-octane sex positivity."
**—Ian Kerner, PhD, LMFT, *New York Times*
bestselling author of *She Comes First***

"The sex-positive tool kit that will transform how you feel about your body and in the bedroom. Amy and April have masterfully created a guide to help you shed the shame and claim the pleasure, passion, and confidence you desire!"
—Dr. Jolene Brighten, NMD, FABNE, author of *Is This Normal?*

"In a culture both obsessed with and ashamed of what happens in the bedroom, *Shameless Sex* unwinds the tangled beliefs that surround sex in the modern age. It's vulnerable, practical, and wise. This guide will help you and your partner transform your beliefs, practices, and mindsets around sex."
—Nate Klemp, PhD, coauthor of *The 80/80 Marriage*

"Get ready to embark on a wild and educational ride with this book! Written by two witty and insightful women, this charming sex and relationship advice book will have you laughing, learning, and loving well. Packed with tips, tricks, and tantalizing tales, it's a must-read for anyone looking to spice up their love life with a touch of gal-pal wisdom and humor."
**—Midori, renowned sexologist, educator, and author
of *The Seductive Art of Japanese Bondage***

"The only shame in *Shameless Sex* is NOT reading this book, and missing out on Amy and April's joyfully curated pleasure paths. Come feel inspired by all the insight they've slipped between two covers, then discover the new erotic pleasures coming your way!"
—Dr. Sadie Allison, author of *Tickle His Pickle*

"While there are some universal truths, there is no one-size-fits-all approach to having a pleasurable, shame-free sex life. Amy and April get that, and in *Shameless Sex*, they provide you with all the tools needed so *you* can figure out and *own* your relationship with sex, no matter how it may look."
**—Zachary Zane, sex columnist and author of
*Boyslut: A Memoir and Manifesto***

"*Shameless Sex* is a timely guide that challenges societal stigmas and encourages readers to embrace their sexuality without shame. By boldly discussing common concerns, fears, and taboos surrounding sexuality in a compassionate and non-judgmental manner, *Shameless Sex* empowers individuals to prioritize their well-being and lift the stigmas associated with sexual health."
—Peter Castillo, MD, founder of Swan Medical Intimate Wellness

SHAMELESS
SEX

Choose Your Own
Pleasure Path to Unlock
the Sex Life You've Been
Waiting For

AMY BALDWIN and
APRIL LAMPERT

BenBella Books, Inc.
Dallas, TX

BenBella Books, Inc.
10440 N. Central Expressway
Suite 800
Dallas, TX 75231
benbellabooks.com
Send feedback to feedback@benbellabooks.com

BenBella is a federally registered trademark.

Printed in the United States of America
10 9 8 7 6 5 4 3 2 1

Library of Congress Control Number: 2023016162
ISBN (hardcover) 9781637743768
ISBN (electronic) 9781637743775

Editing by Leah Baxter and Leah Wilson
Copyediting by Scott Calamar
Proofreading by Jenny Bridges and W. Brock Foreman
Indexing by WordCo Indexing Services
Text design and composition by PerfecType, Nashville, TN
Illustrations by Glen Colligan and Stacey Schwiesow
Cover design by Brigid Pearson
Cover image © Shutterstock / SKT Studio
Printed by Lake Book Manufacturing

Dedicated to YOU (yes, you) and your journey towards having the shameless sex you desire and the pleasure that you deserve, because it's your birthright.

Contents

CONTENTS

shame·less

adjective

(of a person or their conduct) characterized
by or showing a lack of shame.
"My dog is absolutely shameless when he begs."

sex

noun

sexual activity, including sexual intercourse.
"They just had great sex."

shame·less sex

noun

knowing and tending to your sexual needs and boundaries,
speaking your truth and asking for what you want in sex and
relationships, and—as long as you are abiding by consent—
giving zero fucks about what other people think.
"Look at you glowing after all of that shameless sex."

Introduction

How's your bedroom action? Are you having the time of your life between the sheets . . . or not? What if you could have the ultimate pleasure you've been waiting for? What would it be like to have sex and intimacy that goes beyond your wildest imagination? Don't be shy—dare to think big, be fearless, and envision yourself as a liberated sexual being. How would your life be different if you embraced your sexuality and wild freedom? If you were given the key to unlock your ultimate desires and have erotically shameless sex, would you use it? If you're ready to take the plunge, come with us and let us be your guide on your journey toward *Shameless Sex*.

WHAT IS *SHAMELESS SEX*?

Shameless Sex is a map to guide you into living your most authentic and vibrant sexual self to help you unlock the pleasure you hold within. We're Amy and April, sex and relationship experts, co-hosts of the *Shameless Sex* podcast, and best friends with a passion for educating and initiating shame-free conversations about sexuality. *Shameless Sex* is real talk about sex and relationships with a playful twist. We're not afraid to tell it

1

like it is and unabashedly talk about all the facets of sexual pleasure along the way, to help you feel normal, whole, and supported in your journey. *Shameless Sex* encompasses the ever-changing world of sexual pleasure and partnership, as well as the unique challenges that are part of being a human on planet Earth. We strive to normalize all expressions of consensual sex, and we hope to inspire the same in you.

Since 2017, we have released weekly podcast episodes highlighting the vast and ever-changing body of current research, perspectives, and beliefs about sex and relationships. We're on a mission to teach you how to have hotter sex, deeper intimacy, and how to make your own rules for who you are as a sexual being.

THE BIRTH OF *SHAMELESS SEX*

Our podcast journey began in January 2017. We were both freshly out of relationships and had been invited to be guests on our friend Dr. Emily Morse's podcast, *Sex with Emily*. During the interview, we each began sharing some of our sexual adventures, fully unleashing our shameless selves with authenticity. Emily and her producer were laughing uncontrollably most of the show, and that episode—titled "Orgasms, Squirting, and the Year of Anal Licking"—was featured in Emily's "Interview Orgy" mash-up because it was one of her favorite episodes of 2017. A few days after the interview, feeling charged up by our on-air dynamic, we decided to create a podcast together, hoping to inspire others and normalize conversations around sex by sharing our experiences.

We called this collaboration *Shameless Sex*. Though we started small, planning to release only five episodes, we loved every minute of recording and began receiving glowing reviews and even questions from listeners. As the weeks passed, episode downloads only increased, and we knew we had found our life's calling.

As of 2023, the podcast has hundreds of episodes, with a new release every Tuesday. *Shameless Sex* is one of the most listened to podcasts on the globe, consistently ranking between #2 and #4 in the sexuality category and is in the top 1 percent of all podcasts in the world. But as the daily appreciation emails from listeners attest, *Shameless Sex* is so much more than a podcast—or, now, a book. *Shameless Sex* is a sex and relationship revolution. So get ready, because it's time to revolutionize your sexuality and become a sexual shooting star.

ABOUT US—AMY AND APRIL

Amy Baldwin is a sex and relationship coach trained in both the Somatica and Hakomi Methods, a certified sex educator, lead educator for über-lube, and the co-owner of the mother-daughter-owned online pleasure boutique PurePleasureShop.com. April Lampert is the chief sales and partnerships officer and co-owner of Hot Octopuss, an innovative and award-winning sex toy company, and has been educating people about sexual pleasure, health and wellness, and sex toys on a global scale since 2008. We have dedicated our lives to the business of sexual pleasure and relationships. But it's taken both of us a long time to get here.

Amy's Journey as a Sexual Being

I'm a self-proclaimed wounded healer who grew up in the progressive city of Santa Cruz, California. While Santa Cruz felt advanced in sexual politics, I only received very general sex education in school, which left out important information about pleasure in sex. I never learned about orgasm, how to ask for what I wanted, how to advocate for my body, or how to pleasure my body in a way that could work for me. Like most, I had to find out through trial and error during sexual experiences.

I was fortunate enough to grow up in a household with parents who—each in their own ways—let me know sex was not shameful. My dad's contribution was to stay out of my dating and sex life entirely, which was both a blessing, because he did not shame me, and a challenge, because I didn't have a primary masculine figure educating or supporting me. My mom, however, was my saving grace and showed up with everything she could to love me unconditionally, teach me about my intellectual and emotional worthiness, and educate me about sex at a very young age. Not only did she lovingly tell me I could come to her if I wanted to get on birth control, she also gave me a copy of the book *Our Bodies, Ourselves*, and even scheduled my first gynecological visit before I was sexually active.

I finally decided to become sexually active (specifically, to have pene-trative penis-in-vagina—or PIV—sex) at the age of sixteen, and my mom helped me get a prescription for birth control in preparation. My first PIV partner was also my first high school boyfriend. It was new to both of us, and we talked about it many times beforehand. But as is the case for many vulva owners having penetrative sex for the first time, it did not feel pleasurable at all when it actually happened—nor did it on the second or third time. It was uncomfortable, sometimes painful, and confusing—because, I thought, *Isn't sex supposed to feel good?* I felt emotional pleasure being desired and touched by my partner, but I did not enjoy having a penis inside of me. At first, I concluded that it was probably just the way anatomy worked. Thankfully, I realized I was wrong as I immersed myself in learning more about my body and my pleasure.

Considering my rocky start, how did I get into the field of helping people have better, more authentic, and fulfilling sex and relationships? One of my biggest inspirations was my first college human sexuality class. I was eighteen and barely understood my body. I had been intimate with multiple partners, yet I had only experienced orgasm from my first vibrator. Needless to say, I had a lot of questions and no idea where to go or who to ask, so taking a human sexuality class seemed like the perfect place to start.

Though the professor was dull and passionless, I somehow found myself loving every minute of it. Even after studying disturbing images of sexually transmitted infections/sexually transmitted diseases (or STIs/STDs) in the textbooks and sitting through endless dry lectures, I couldn't get enough. Not only were my personal questions getting answered, but I also felt a sense of fulfillment. The more material I consumed, the more I *knew* that I was meant to work in the field of sex-positive education.

I went on to major in psychology with a minor in human sexuality at San Francisco State University and planned to move into the field of sex therapy. But during a sex-ed class field trip, a visit to one of San Francisco's premier boutique sex shops changed my direction entirely. The store was clean, comfortable, and welcoming. Customers were invited to touch and feel the sensations of each product on display to find something to fit their unique needs. The staff acted as attentive guides and teachers, helping customers along and explaining how to use and care for each toy. This store even had weekly workshops like Toy Safety, Anal Sex How-Tos, and Oral Sex 101. Through education without shame or stigma, they were helping people bring more pleasure into their lives.

After this trip, I kept returning to the idea of opening a store like that in Santa Cruz. Coincidentally, my mom was looking for a business investment at the time, so I quickly called her. I described the sex shop, and said, "Mom, we don't have anything like that at home, and they're really helping people. We should open a sex shop together." She was surprised but intrigued. Her response was "Me? A sex shop?"

Two years later, in 2008, my mom and I opened the doors to Pure Pleasure Shop. We wanted to focus on facilitating a safe, welcoming, shame-free experience no matter what our customers were interested in—especially since many people would walk through the front door with a fair amount of fear or shame about seeking sex advice or product guidance. Everything from the legitimacy of the products we recommended to staff's attitudes and language all mattered, and we dedicated time to educating ourselves and the staff to speak inclusively and without judgment.

It was this, along with the desire to teach pleasure-based workshops, that led me to my next move: becoming a certified sex educator through San Francisco Sex Information's intensive training program. I then went on to complete Barbara Carrellas's Urban Tantra Professional Training Program as well. Next, I decided I wanted to learn how to work with people on their sex and relationship issues one-on-one and signed up for an intensive sex and relationship coaching training program through Somatica. Not only did this give me the skills to work with individuals in my own private practice, but it also taught me about myself—including how to advocate for my needs and boundaries, how to tap into my ultimate erotic self, and how to handle and heal ruptures in relationships. It was life changing.

I attribute much of the creation of *Shameless Sex* to my experience in Somatica. In fact, it was in that training I met Dr. Emily Morse, which led to the beginning of my on-air collaboration with April Lampert, my best friend and fellow sex toy industry mogul. Speaking of which—let's meet April.

April's Sexuality Evolution

I have a BS in environmental law and policy from the University of Minnesota, Twin Cities, and an insatiable appetite for changing the world. I grew up in a small town in Wisconsin in a blue-collar, conservative household. No one ever talked about sex growing up, and I only knew of my genitals as my "no-no" zone—you don't touch it, and you don't show it to others, ever. The first time I heard the word "sex," I was in kindergarten, and a girl at school asked me, "Do you like sex?" I had no idea what sex was, but I assumed it was some kind of food. That night at the dinner table I asked my brother, "Can you pass me the ketchup and some sex?" My mom lost it, pulling me off my chair and dragging me to my room while screaming that I should *never* utter that word again. I assumed it was another bad word like "fuck" or "shit," so I complied and didn't say that word aloud until many years later.

Fast-forward to my first year of high school. I had zero idea what sex with someone else should be like, but I loved how masturbation made me feel—although I believed it was wrong, and it left me with a strong sense of guilt every time. I started dating a much-older high school senior with a tough-guy persona and long history of being a womanizer. (Spoiler alert: this relationship would yield my first traumatic sexual experience.) I wanted to impress him, but I was also adamant about waiting until I was sixteen to go "all the way" with him. At first, he was fine with some handjobs, fingering, and kissing, but after a few weeks of only this type of play, he requested a blowjob. I had never given anyone a blowjob before, and I was terrified. But one night, during our typical fully clothed, heavy make-out session, he took off his pants and boxers. He started pushing my head down between his legs, telling me I should "give it a little kiss, just one. Come on, I have blue balls and you gotta do something about it." He then began forcefully thrusting his hips into my face so his penis was touching my lips, trying to pry my mouth open as I resisted.

After this incident, sex and relationships became very confusing to me. I went down a dark and insecure path, having a lot of compliant sex, faking orgasms so I could get sex over with, and never speaking to my needs during sexual experiences because I believed they didn't matter. I convinced myself that only a man should orgasm during sex, and that my orgasms should only happen in secret through masturbation. This was my sexual life until my late twenties.

No one at home or in school ever educated me on sex or pleasure. In high school, sex education was centered around human anatomy, a video of childbirth, abstinence, and two terrible examples of how to put a condom on a banana. That was it. Nothing about pleasure or consent or safer sex. And if you got an STI or became pregnant, your life was over and your future ruined. If any students were brave enough to ask questions during these classes, they were bullied for days afterward. These sex-ed classes only drove my insecurities, fear, and shame deeper. Sex reverted to that bad word I had uttered at the dinner table so many years before, and I began to think my mom was right. Sex is a terrible thing, so I should probably erase it from my mind entirely.

Considering my history, you may be wondering what inspired me to enter the field of sexuality. Well, it was a total accident. In my early twenties, my best friend Amy was opening a sex shop with her mother in Santa Cruz, California, where I was living at the time, and she convinced me to work there as a store manager. I had never set foot inside a sex shop, and I'd never even seen—let alone used—a vibrator before. I *never* talked about sex, because I carried a ton of shame around it. I thought Amy was a bit crazy for thinking I would be the right fit, but after some convincing, I finally agreed. And she was right—it turns out that my lack of shyness, ability to connect with people, and openness to learning made me very good at speaking to people about their pleasure. Working at Pure Pleasure Shop opened a door for me. I became enthralled with the world of sexuality. I started reading as many books about sex as I could find, and I tested new vibrators every week. I educated myself on the right language to use so I could be as sex positive as possible and attended Pure Pleasure's sex-ed workshops. Amy and I would also attend sex toy trade shows so I could check out new products with her. I finally began to feel a sense of sexual freedom and openness—and yet I still carried my shame around because I didn't have the tools I needed to heal myself.

It was at one of these trade shows I met the (former) CEO of Fun Factory USA, a German manufacturer known for making some of the best-quality toys in the industry. He asked if I would be interested in working their booth at future trade shows and, two trade shows later, he offered me a full-time sales position. My life became immersed in all things sexual pleasure. I was educating people about sex toys, the diversity of the human body, inclusive language, manufacturing practices, and sex toy materials and lubricants, and I traveled all over the world for trainings and to help with product development. Six years after my start at Fun Factory, I saw how much Hot Octopuss was changing people's lives, and I brought my expertise there in order to be a part of something bigger. Not long after, Amy and I started our passion-project-turned-global-phenomenon *Shameless Sex*. I never thought in a million years that this conservative Midwestern girl with a wildly shame-filled past could end up here. But in the most unorthodox way possible, my dreams of changing the world have become an incredible reality.

HOW TO USE THIS BOOK

Over the years, the *Shameless Sex* podcast has received countless sex and relationship questions. After answering these inquiries, we realized that almost all of them revolved around one (or more) of the same general concerns. It became clear that most people, no matter their age, gender, or relationship status, are facing different versions of the same sexual and relational issues. *Am I (or is this) normal? Am I broken? How can I learn to become a better lover? How can I spice up my sex life with more passion and connection? How can I talk to my partner about what I want sexually, or how do I even discover what I want in the first place?*

This book is designed to be navigated like a map to help you find your way to fulfilling your personal needs, desires, and understanding around relationships and sexuality. Many relationship self-help books offer solutions without teaching readers the complexities of sexuality, but we don't want to help you paper over your problems or concerns—we want to help you explore and address every part of yourself. *Shameless Sex* realizes that humans have many layers, and what is perceived from the outside is only a fraction of the whole person. By peeling back every layer, you can reveal and process the deep complexities and shadows that exist within yourself.

Not only will *Shameless Sex* offer you the modern perspectives and advice of educators, authors, doctors, therapists, coaches, podcasters, and everyday people we've interviewed on our podcast, but it will also help you discover our unique formula for uncovering different options, or *Pleasure Paths*, that will lead you to other chapters that focus on the practices and tools that you'll need to reach the outcomes you desire.

This book was intentionally organized with the not-so-shiny and heavier stuff first. The reason is that it's more effective to work toward resolving any hidden complexities first so that they don't later block you from unlocking sexual mastery. If you're on the path to achieve this, then you can't stick a shame Band-Aid on it before moving on to the playful stuff.

If you find yourself wanting to skip certain chapters because the topics seem less appealing, that's understandable. But consider how building a house—especially if it's the house of your dreams—without a strong foundation makes it vulnerable to falling apart when difficult conditions are at hand. Although difficulties are an inevitable part of sex and relationships, you can still work to have mind-blowing orgasms, limitless pleasure, great communication, and lots of shameless sex.

If you were born before 1998, you may remember Choose Your Own Adventure books, in which you, the reader, are presented with a situation and a set of choices and are invited to use your imagination to navigate the story and achieve your desired ending. *Shameless Sex* offers a similar approach. But in this book, you're not trying to photograph an abominable snowman or discover the lost city of Atlantis, because this book applies to your life. Real life. It's for YOU, the sexually inquisitive and adventurous human who wants to take the bull by the horns and make their own rules for sex and relationships. Unless otherwise noted, the reader has no gender, sexual orientation, or relationship style—because this book is written for everyone. Each chapter contains sex questions pertaining to the chapter's title followed by a section called "Choose Your Own Pleasure Path" (or CYOPP), with various options you can choose from to achieve the outcomes you desire.

Every Choose Your Own Adventure book starts with the disclaimer: "You and you alone are in charge of what happens in this story . . . At any time YOU can go back and make another choice, alter the path of your story, and change your result." Similarly, in this book you are also in control of your outcome, and you will need to apply the skills you learn here to get the results you're looking for. But this story is yours, so you can go back at any time and choose another Pleasure Path if you'd like to explore a new or different direction.

Throughout this book, you will find a plethora of tips, tools, and techniques inspired by the most common sex questions the *Shameless Sex* podcast has received. You'll also find podcast episode references, giving you additional resources to dive deeper into scenarios that you relate to. While much of the book's content requires some level of work and dedication, why add more stress to your life trying to figure out a problem when there are pathways to applicable solutions laid out for you throughout each chapter? Even though some of the nuances of a particular sex question may not seem like they are part of your story or individual vision, we recommend considering carefully before skipping over them, as they may still be relevant to you in some way.

If this sounds scary or like too much of an undertaking, or if some of the most common sex questions are not resonating with you at this point in your life, that's fine. Because guess what? This book will be waiting for you like a stage-five clinger, forever lingering on the sidelines to take you down the path toward having the sex and relationships that you want, when you want them. While we hope you will live in a world full of sexy sunshine and racy rainbows, *Shameless Sex* has you covered if or when you encounter storms, because it's designed to be revisited time and time again.

Are you willing to make the leap? Ready to open yourself up by being vulnerable and proactive so you can create the lasting change in the sex and relationships you desire? *Shameless Sex* applauds you and your immense courage, strength, and fearlessness—you are a total badass human being! While the road ahead may be rocky and even treacherous at times, the rewards will be massive as you begin to experience the passion, richness, depth, and connection possible in your sex and relationship(s). Thank you for diving into yourself, for doing this hard work, for initiating the change you want to see in your life, and for taking charge of your future self. Thank you for being part of the *Shameless Sex* revolution.

The *Shameless Sex* Philosophy

We shared in the introduction how essential it is to be in charge of your own sexual journey, especially when it comes to making any lasting change. As you read each chapter of this book, you will notice that we never offer a quick fix or a generic one-size-fits-all approach to solving the challenges at hand. Instead, we encourage you as an individual to become an active participant in reprogramming your approach to sex and relationships.

However, there are a few general philosophies that carry through every aspect of our work. We want to clearly define these fundamental principles for you because they will provide strong guidance on your sexual journey. Consider these the *Shameless Sex* Bill of Rights because they are elemental to this book (and to life itself!).

ALWAYS START WITH CONSENT AND SAFETY

"Consent" is a buzzword that's thrown around a lot—and for good reason. It's generally defined as permission for something to happen or an agreement to do something. But it's so much more than that. To paraphrase Rainn.org's definition, it's an agreement between participants to engage in sexual activity where it is **actively**, **clearly**, and **freely** communicated. This requires an affirmative verbal expression where everyone involved in the sexual experience fully understands each other's boundaries.

Consent requires a conscious mind that is coherent and not intoxicated—in other words, capable of making autonomous choices. Coerced consent is not consent. Consent requires a moment in time when all adults involved can check in with themselves and openly express their yes, no, or maybe another time.

It's amazing what can happen when consent is presented and upheld throughout a sexual experience. Amy, a self-proclaimed hater of most ticklish sensations, can attest to the power of consent and safety through a life-changing experience involving her armpit and a sexy cuddle puddle.

Amy was newly single, recovering from heartbreak, feeling disconnected from her sexual essence, and highly protective of her body. She actively chose to be in a sexually charged environment with people who were new to her. Before things got hot and heavy, one of the participants of the cuddle puddle checked in with Amy, saying something along the lines of, "How are you feeling? I'm curious what your boundaries and needs are." This inspired Amy to share that she needed to take things slow, that her pants would stay on, and her genitals were off the table. Her boundaries were respected, and everyone continued to check in with each other along the way. The pussy-throbbing magic that ensued resulted in a night that not only recharged her sex drive, but also gave her a newfound love for armpit-gasms.

This form of high-level consent allowed Amy's entire being to fully relax as she knew her yeses, nos, and maybes—as well as those of all participants—were of the utmost importance. In the safety of the cuddle puddle, she made the embodied choice to allow one person's mouth to find its way to her armpit, and what began as a tickle transformed into an overwhelming sensation of intense pleasure. She discovered her armpits to be another mind-blowing erogenous zone on her body, and she learned a deep lesson about the importance of active and continuously negotiated consent as a means toward safe sexual exploration and even immense pleasure and orgasm.

YOU SHOULD STOP SHOULD-ING YOURSELF

Forget everything you were told about how sex and relationships *should* be. What you crave sexually matters, and as long as you are behaving safely and conscientiously toward others, there's no reason to waste your time on external expectations that don't align with your intrinsic desires.

We know this can be hard. If you're a human living in the world, you've probably been inundated with sexuality "shoulds" and "shouldn'ts." *You should save sex for committed relationships, you should want sex all the time, your arousal should always correspond to your desire, you (and your partner) should always orgasm during sex, you should only be with one person for the rest of your life,* and *you should only be attracted to the "opposite" sex,* to name a few. And then there's the shouldn'ts: *You shouldn't have sex with too many people, you shouldn't want to have sex with someone other than your partner, you shouldn't engage in "dirty" or taboo sexual behaviors, you shouldn't talk about sex . . .* the list goes on and on.

April lived in a world where sexual expression was always expected to adhere to a particular norm. She discovered how great masturbation felt at a very young age, but since she was shamed for touching herself, she went through life thinking it was wrong—feeling guilty every time self-pleasure resulted in orgasm, something she still works on overcoming to this day. In addition, she was attracted to multiple genders but was told by peers and parents that she should only have interest in one sex—specifically, penis owners. When she entered a relationship with someone of the same sex at the age of nineteen, she hid it and lied about it, shamefully believing society as well as her friends and family would think she was a terrible person and fearing their judgment.

Learning to free herself from the pressure of expectations like these has made her life immeasurably better—and more pleasurable. When she finally learned in her late twenties that masturbation was totally normal and even healthy for her, she was excited. But she was even more amazed to learn that sexual orientation is a spectrum, not a binary, and that sexual attraction doesn't have to be either/or—or even stay the same over time. Knowing that sex doesn't have to live in a world of shoulds and shouldn'ts has brought more peace, love, and yumminess to her sexual experiences than she ever thought possible. Let this be your last should from this point on: you should stop should-ing yourself! Pinky swear, sex gets better when you don't.

THERE'S NOTHING WRONG WITH YOU

Humans are byproducts of their environment and experiences. From anatomy to internal programming, physiology to genealogy, even location and habits—all can have an impact on sexual programming. It's important to recognize that pleasure is pleasure no matter how it presents, and orgasm happens in a multitude of ways, even if it's not what you had anticipated or assumed. Neither the outside world nor a sexual partner's needs determine what your pleasure should be or who you are as a sexual being. And if you have even an inkling of an *I'm not good enough* or *Something's wrong with me* mentality, no matter the reason, it's time to change that story line. These negative beliefs are NEVER true, and it's time you recognize that they were never yours to begin with—they're often born from the same shoulds and shouldn'ts that we tossed in the garbage a page or so ago.

To this day, April continues to have challenges in certain aspects of sex and relationships. She still gets stuck in her head during partnered sexual experiences. She also struggles with slowing down. Her pace in daily life is very fast, so it's difficult to change that in the bedroom. These things don't at all reflect April's inherent worth, only her life experiences. And because she's become aware of them, she is also able to address them. She continuously works at being present and feeling the sensations in her body as well as making shifts to lower her speed during sexual encounters. It's difficult to break old patterns ingrained into your system, but it can be done.

Your brain's complex programming affords you the ability to learn infinite ways to build connection and pleasure. It can even free you from the shackles of past shame and trauma. Yes, it will probably take some work to reboot and reprogram your system, but YOU are worth it.

THE BRAIN IS YOUR LARGEST SEX ORGAN

Imagine the scene. You are sitting down with Amy and April, sipping a tasty beverage, and pondering a question they just posed: What is the most powerful sex organ in your body?

Suddenly, the classic melody from *Jeopardy!* begins to play in the background while you contemplate—Do do do do, do do dooo. Do do do do DUT, dut do do do do . . . Have your answer?

If you hadn't cheated and looked at the subheading, you might respond as many people do, with an answer like the skin, heart, mouth, or the most obvious of choices, the genitals. And these are all great answers, yet none are correct. The connection between all these body parts and their functioning is . . . the brain! Your brain holds primary responsibility for how you view and experience sexuality. It shapes your perception of sex and relationships, including reacting to external societal pressures or personal behavior tendencies. As far as sex goes, your brain is far more powerful and important than any other organ in your entire body.

Hopefully you're shamelessly celebrating your largest sex organ with us because there are some unbelievable takeaway pieces here: the brain is highly malleable, which means that with time, effort, and dedication to your ultimate outcome, you can condition and rewire your brain to experience pleasure and orgasms in ways that you desire—just like those cheesy rom-coms and steamy dramas.

Have you ever had an orgasm in your sleep? Maybe you've woken up feeling like you had a blissful or intense release of some sort. While you're processing the experience, you may realize you never touched your genitals at all. Whether you have or haven't had this superhot, sometimes wet, and ultimately empowering experience, it's a prime example of the capacity the brain has to unleash your sexual pleasure potential, oftentimes unconsciously. Furthermore, "getting fucked" in dreamland can be even hotter than in real life, because your brain is controlling every moment that's unfolding. So bring it on, brain!

But it's not only sexy dreams that can aid in shifting the paradigm for pleasure. Certified sexologist, sex educator, and acclaimed author Barbara Carrellas, along with iconic sexologist, sex educator, and sexual pioneer Annie Sprinkle, PhD, have been teaching people techniques to breathe themselves into orgasm—with zero genital contact—for decades. Furthermore, innovative sex toy company Hot Octopuss used years of medical research and clinical studies of penis owners with spinal cord injuries to develop penis toys that don't require hands, stroking, or erections for a person to reach orgasm. Their line of Guybrators can induce ejaculations even when the penis is flaccid, shifting the outdated paradigm that a penis must be erect to experience sexual pleasure, ejaculate, or orgasm and further exemplifying the immense control the brain has over everyone's pleasure. Now that's a nice load of information!

The idea that orgasm can only occur with genital stimulation is another archaic theory that we happen to know is false. At *Shameless Sex*, we've had (and spoken about) nipple-gasms, ear-gasms, foot-gasms, and even armpit-gasms that resulted in full-body erotic sensation, including pleasure and orgasm. Sometimes these experiences happened randomly or unexpectedly, but when they happened, it was always: 1) in a safe and comfortable space, 2) with a partner who cared about the pleasure they were giving rather than looking to satisfy their own needs, and 3) when we allowed ourselves to get out of our heads and into our bodily sensations. With so many options to achieve orgasm that don't involve the genitals, it's clear that sexual pleasure stems from the brain more than anything else. It's all in your head, honey.

CHANGE ONLY HAPPENS WHEN YOU CHANGE

Change starts with you! Giving all of yourself to a particular story line or belief, whether new or old, *can* become your reality. After all, your ever-changing brain is your largest sex organ. If your brain can change, then your relationship with sex can too.

For April, *Shameless Sex* has helped sculpt her life into something she never imagined it would be. She has always considered herself a "heady" person, but after developing self-care practices like meditation and breath work, she was able to gain an internal awareness she hadn't tapped into before that directly enhanced her sex life. For most of her adult life, April had a lot of compliant sex, feeling embarrassed to talk about her sexual fantasies and turn-ons, never wanting to be vulnerable with a partner because she thought being vulnerable meant being weak, and she wanted to seem strong and put together. But after implementing the knowledge and tools she's gained from many *Shameless Sex* podcast interviews, she was finally capable of identifying where she was stuck, so she could create practices that shifted her from headedness into embodiment.

This shift has also helped April finally release the judgment she once had for others' sexual proclivities. She stopped pooh-poohing the sexual fantasies of others and fully believes that (if there's consent!) it's okay to desire whatever you want. *Never* again will she yuck someone's yum. Releasing these judgments has been a mechanism of healing for April and has marked a powerful transitional point in her journey toward living a deeply fulfilling and highly pleasurable life.

Within this liberation from the judgment of others, April has also learned how to be more gentle with herself. She has overcome the shame she's carried around for decades (from an STI diagnosis and a scarred outer labium from a teenage sexual incident) by creating awareness, practicing self-compassion, and reframing the narrative anytime that toxic shame attempts to seep back into her life again. Most of all, this pleasure pilgrimage has allowed her to find her true self while giving her the most precious gift of all: purpose. From a very young age, April aspired to change the world for the better and improve the quality of people's lives—though she never imagined talking unashamedly about sex and sharing her experiences would be a means to inspire change to happen. But guess what? Change can and will happen if you initiate and welcome it.

If you approach sexuality with compassion for yourself and your intimate partner(s) and the understanding that YOU are the orchestrator of your own erotic symphony, you can bring yourself ever closer to the sex and relationships you desire.

Let's face it, change is inevitable. Whether solo or partnered, you and your approach to sex can and will evolve—hopefully for the better. Part of improving your approach to sex involves embracing shifts with open arms, while continuously communicating clearly about your needs and desires. Be patient and embrace the way your body uniquely experiences pleasure, even when you hit those proverbial roadblocks. There could be a pot of pleasure at the end of your journey (and that's worth more than a bunch of gold).

CULTIVATE PRESENCE—GO SLOWER THAN SLOW, THEN SLOWER THAN THAT

Public service announcement! Take it from the two heady, fast-moving individuals writing this: things are a lot easier when you slow the fuck down. This includes everything from the actions you take to the ways you communicate and think, as well as the touch you give and receive. After all, how can you fully appreciate and relax into pleasure if you don't give yourself time to enjoy it?

Please meet a good friend who is slightly frustrating yet continuously rewarding you: presence. Being present involves being fully focused on what is occurring within and around you in each moment. There are times when presence isn't helpful, such as situations involving shame, trauma, or sexual violence. But when it comes to the yummy stuff, where there's consensual intimacy and connection with yourself or others, presence is the most precious of all tools in your erotic tool kit. Practicing presence encourages proactive responses to stimulation rather than pre-programmed reactive replies. It also cultivates connectedness with yourself as well as with your surroundings, and it helps your mind focus on what you're doing rather than what you're *not* doing.

Presence requires your complete attention and usually necessitates you to invite its best friend to the party as well (it's not the *Shameless Sex* duo, although Amy and April love a party with lots of presence).

Presence's most complementary ally and ultimate bestie is slowness. As you work toward presence, you will find yourself needing to slow down not just the pace of your physical movements but also the pace of your thoughts and decisions. By being intentional with yourself, you can tap into presence and slowness in both your mind and body. One will follow the other. To initiate a slowdown, ask yourself questions like: *What am I feeling now? What am I desiring? Where do I need more boundaries?*

Amy can attest to the efficacy of presence through slowness because it changed her sex life completely. When she was in her early twenties, the sex she was having was pretty transactional, and she lived by the motto "I don't make love; I fuck." It was always fast and not very intimate—until a profound sexual encounter changed all of that. Instead of fucking, Amy and her lover slowly explored new and titillating sensations, connecting with each other deeply. Three hours felt like an eternity of sensual bliss where nothing else mattered besides each decadent skin-to-skin touch. Through presence and slowness, Amy discovered she enjoyed and was exceptionally proficient at making love as well as fucking. This is just one example of why we constantly advocate for slowing down and why our ultimate *Shameless Sex* motto is: *Go slower than slow, then slower than that*, because "It really works!"

YOUR FIRST SEXUAL RELATIONSHIP IS WITH YOU

Finally, the most powerful sexual experiences are the ones that you have engineered yourself. Whether you're single or in a relationship, when you're in charge of your own sexual experiences—alone or with someone else—you'll find that you are able to own and enjoy your sexuality in a way you never could before. The best thing about having a sexual relationship with yourself is that you can always make it better. It can be hard to have an intense and fulfilling sex life when you're in a long-term relationship or involved with a partner who doesn't share the same sexual desires, tastes, or fantasies as you do. That's why it's important that *you* find what works for *you* and make adjustments accordingly as you go along. By practicing the principles outlined in these pages, you will learn how to have better sex and more fulfilling relationships. If you're ready to take the next steps and make real changes in your sexual life, then turn the page and let the shameless adventure begin.

Am I Normal?

The fear of not being "normal" is at the core of almost *all* the sex questions we receive at *Shameless Sex*. While the actual question may not even contain the word "normal," the underlying inquiry about feeling different or inadequate remains: *Why do I desire sex and relationships in this way when other people are having different experiences? Is it okay that my desire conflicts with my partner's? Why doesn't my body do what I think it should during sex? Are the ways I desire pleasure wrong? Are the ways I want to connect in my relationships okay? Am I the only one who feels this way?*

Feeling *not normal* might leave you with a sense of aloneness and powerlessness, as though you're incapable or unworthy of having the sex and relationships you desire and the pleasure you deserve. But *Shameless Sex* is here to tell you there *is* no normal, especially when it comes to human sexuality. And whatever you're struggling with, you aren't alone—trust us, someone else out there has struggled with it too.

Shameless Sex has a motto for anyone who's ever felt like an outcast, alone, weird, different, or abnormal in their sexuality: Normal is boring as fuck! Yes, we may all be a little different—but at least we're not all the same.

THERE'S NOTHING DYSFUNCTIONAL ABOUT YOU

Human beings have a lot in common with each other: Everyone comes from the same embryological design, everyone's body changes over time, and everyone needs breath, water, and food to survive. Other than this, there is little common ground to define what constitutes a "normal" human being. In other words, unless you have figured out the magical art of breatharianism, you are *completely normal* and there is nothing wrong with you.

In her revolutionary book *Come As You Are: The Surprising New Science That Will Transform Your Sex Life*, Emily Nagoski, PhD, examines the science behind human development in utero and how all humans have the same tissues, just arranged in different ways, with infinite variety in function and appearance. For instance, the head of the penis is embryologically the same tissue as that of the clitoris and, just like the clitoris, is responsible for the majority of sensation for sexual pleasure. And while some general trends are observed—for example, most people with XY chromosomes develop penises and most people with XX develop vulvas—that's certainly not the end of it. Other people develop genitalia that are not within the confines of the current socially constructed penis-and-vagina binary. And even within these broad categories, your genitals are as unique as your fingerprints, with no one else in the world having the exact same contours and ridges as you.

Not to mention the individuality of your DNA, personality traits, environment, and likes and dislikes. There really is only one YOU on the planet, and the way you relate to others is exclusive to you. Considering all of this, it becomes apparent the only thing that's normal about being a human is being different. Yet anyone who doesn't fit into some fictitious standard of sexuality still faces external stigma and, often, internal feelings of inadequacy.

 Emily Nagoski shares her expertise, research, and some life-changing knowledge in Episode #95, "Come as You Are Because YES, You Are Normal."

The criteria for normalcy are based on socially constructed ideas about what is common or appropriate here and now. This means it's entirely contextual and shifts based on time, place, or other people's opinions. The standard for "normal" sexual behavior greatly differs from California to Brazil to Mozambique, and it will likely change in the years to come. In our opinion, this is highly problematic. What an arbitrary thing to judge someone for. And yet, people do—all the time. Society's constant worry about being "normal" likely stems from the shame others may have projected on them as to how they should or should not be.

KEEP YOUR ENEMIES CLOSE, INCLUDING SHAME

When lovers, parents, or peers criticize you, it can plant a seed of shame that alters your perception of your identity—and, eventually, impacts your sense of self throughout your life. Shame exists entirely in relation to others and hinges on your sense of belonging (or not) in your family, friend circle, lovership, or community. Perhaps someone expressed disapproval or disappointment about your sexual performance, and you felt inadequate and unworthy. Or someone made an observation about your body, and you got the impression you were different from everyone else, and that there was something wrong with you. This shame can become a deeply rooted part of you, tainting your self-image and undermining positive views about yourself. It can also adversely impact your relationships by fueling conflict and twisting a partner's neutral comments into reinforcements of any previously felt inadequacies—provoking defensiveness, sadness, anger, and emotional shutdown.

The effects of shame are a perfect example of the sexual power of the brain because it can inhibit pleasure, but, crucially, it can also transform your connection to it. You *can* work with shame and rediscover sexual fulfillment.

The prospect of such a big change can be downright terrifying, so if you're feeling some resistance to the process, know you're not alone. But trust us, the rewards are worth it. Remind yourself of this every time self-doubt, insecurity, or resistance kicks in. This is an opportunity to let go of what no longer serves you while embracing your true desires.

Can you imagine living in an alternate universe where not one person will judge you for the way you live your life, including the way you express yourself as a sexual being? How would you live your life knowing it was entirely safe to be the true, authentic you?

SHAMELESS SEX IS WITH YOU

Both Amy and April have experienced those feelings of being "not normal" and different from others throughout our sexual histories. We first learned how to "do" sex from mainstream media, religion, peers, and porn, all of which taught the same reductive, cis-heteronormative bullshit: that PIV sex is the only way, and that it should always be a certain way (usually, between a cisgender man who holds all the sexual agency and cums first and a cisgender woman who puts her pleasure last, if it's considered at all). From our experience, having those expectations became extra problematic because neither of us could orgasm from PIV sex alone, causing sex to be focused around putting the penis owner's pleasure before our own. This further instilled the sense of being abnormal and problematic because we were expected to want to put our pleasure last. Expectations like these continue to systemically alter people's sexual experiences across many generations.

In a Dark Room with the Bloodhound Gang

Amy initially encountered the feeling of being sexually "abnormal" when someone other than herself touched her genitals for the first time. She was in her freshman year of high school, at a cozy gathering where everyone started coupling up and making out. She paired up with a seemingly disinterested boy she barely knew and ended up in a dark room alone with him. Without any connection or warm-up, he put his hands down her pants and fingered her, while the Bloodhound Gang's

"The Bad Touch" played in the background. Needless to say, the song—*You and me, baby, ain't nothin' but mammals, so let's do it like they do on the Discovery Channel (Gettin' horny now)*—did not enhance the touch. In fact, it felt uncomfortable—almost painful. Amy was confused, as she was under the impression that sexual touch in erogenous zones should conjure pleasurable sensations. So why didn't this feel good? Plenty of her friends said they enjoyed having their genitals touched. She thought: *Is there something wrong with me? Is my body different from other girls'?*

It wasn't until her early twenties, after a fair amount of self-exploration and pleasurable sexual experiences with others, that Amy's doubt disappeared. She learned that her body needed time, slowness, and enjoyed specific variations of touch far from the classic finger bang. Her mind desired connection, safety, and a feeling of being cared for. With the help of thoughtful lovers, years of sex education, and the power of her own two hands, Amy discovered what turns her on and embraced the unique ways she experiences pleasure knowing fully: *No, there is nothing wrong with me. Yes, I am normal. And I'm giving finger banging the middle finger.*

April and Her Beloved Teddy Bear, Barry

April discovered masturbation at six, when she learned how to hump her favorite teddy bear, Barry. She regularly rubbed her "no-no" zone on Barry's stuffed nose until she experienced an intense release inside her body. She did this so often that Barry's nose began to flatten and a white crust developed, forcing her to wash Barry's face in the sink regularly to avoid her mother's questioning. Even though April had absolutely no idea what masturbation or orgasm was at that time, she knew that it felt good to hump her stuffed bear—and that it wasn't something she should share with anyone else. She believed it was "bad" and made her very different from all the other kids.

Later, at the age of eight, April accidentally stumbled upon gang-bang porn on a videotape mislabeled as her mother's favorite soap opera. Until the tape disappeared months later, she watched it repeatedly, humping her teddy bear surreptitiously. After this, her lust for new masturbation material was fervent enough that she scoured every forbidden videotape in her house, especially those rated PG-13 or R, until she had developed a collection of the hottest sex scenes from movies like *Pretty Woman*, *Dirty Dancing*, *Top Gun*, and *Fatal Attraction* (her absolute favorite because you could almost see Michael Douglas's penis as he penetrates Glenn Close in the stove-top sex scene).

April convinced herself that all sex and relationships should look like those movies. This generated a lot of issues for her once she started getting physical with boys in her teenage years. She had become so accustomed to closeted masturbation that when she started having real sexual experiences with boys (kissing, touching, breast fondling, and fingering), it was far from pleasurable or sexy. It was uncomfortable and awkward, and she was always in her head thinking about when the physical part would be over. And when it was over, she was left confused as to why none of it was like the movies. She convinced herself she must be different from everyone else. She must be a weirdo and fucked up. If she wasn't getting pleasure from being touched by others, something had to be wrong with her.

It took April twenty-seven years to finally realize she wasn't some sexual outcast. While working at Pure Pleasure Shop, she finally had a safe environment to gather information about sex from people and resources she trusted. She attended sex-ed workshops and learned that you should talk about your sexual yeses, nos, and maybes before and even during sex. She was shocked to discover that her sexual needs mattered just as much as her partner's, and that it wasn't her job to please her partner, either. She also learned that several of her vulva-owning coworkers had never orgasmed from penetrative sex. She was fueled by discovering she wasn't a weirdo, and she felt more confidence in the bedroom knowing that she wasn't alone—especially when she started using external vibrators during sex to help her reach orgasm, leading to her very first orgasm from PIV sex. From then on, she knew her sex life would never be the same.

TESTI(CLE)MONIALS: BREAKTHROUGHS FOR EMBRACING THE NEW NORMAL

As our personal stories—and countless testimonials from our beloved listeners—confirm, it's actually more normal to feel like you're *not* normal. The following testimonials remind us we are not the only ones battling these internal beliefs, and that with deep inquiry and practice, we can generate immense growth and self-acceptance.

"I just wanted to say how much I enjoyed episode #269, 'Everything We Wished We Knew in Our Teens, 20s, and 30s. I've learned so much from every episode, but this one made me feel normal. I'm an outlier as a male; I don't identify with most of the male generalizations out there, and this episode was more about our individual struggles and the importance of embracing our differences. Thank you and keep up all the good work."

"I love your podcast and want to thank you for helping me overcome shame around my own cis-hetero-male sexuality while better understanding my lover and her sexual experience, and for introducing me to a multitude of other human experiences that I otherwise might not have been open to."

"I love sex but have always had a hard time talking about it. Having now listened to a good number of your podcasts, I am happy to report that I have just managed to have a completely candid and open discussion with my partner without feeling awkward or embarrassed for the first time ever. You've helped me put into words how I feel about my desires and taught me not to be ashamed of my sex drive and kinks."

It bears repeating: Your unique expression as a sexual being is normal and should be celebrated! But also, as long as you want to change for *you*, there's nothing wrong with wanting to shift things in some way. If you are looking to make your sex life more fulfilling, there are a lot of aspects of your beliefs, actions, or behaviors that can help you achieve those goals. Remember how April used to think her need for external stimulation to feel pleasure was a problem, only for it to transition into a life-altering tool in her orgasmic tool kit? Well, guess what? The same can apply to you. Once you embrace what makes you unique, your sexual future is full of so many possibilities.

We would like to issue a disclaimer, though: *Shameless Sex* cannot give medical advice because Amy and April are not MDs. So when the question *Am I normal?* relates to physiology or potential health issues, it's best to consult a trusted medical professional to find the right answers and possible solutions. That said, we'll cover adapting sexually to psychological and bodily changes, as well as other health-based challenges, in Chapter 2 by sharing advice and tips from some phenomenal experts in those areas.

I HAVE A DIFFICULT TIME ORGASMING

I'm in a long-term relationship, and I rarely orgasm from penetrative sex. It drives me crazy. I easily orgasm from clitoral stimulation, and I've tried what feels like everything, but it just never seems to come (pun intended). Is this normal? Are some women not able to orgasm vaginally? Or can I learn how to have orgasms from penetration? Is there anything you can recommend I try?

Questions like this are very common from vulva owners, especially (but not exclusively.) those who are in relationships with penis owners. And we get similar questions from penis owners who feel frustration about their inability to bring vulva-owning partners to orgasm via internal penetration alone (as well as questions about their own challenges with orgasming during certain types of stimulation—hang in there, because that will be addressed in this chapter too).

The Science Behind Vulva Arousal

Let's start by saying: If you've never experienced orgasm from internal vaginal stimulation alone, there is *nothing* wrong with you.

A lot of vulva owners require external stimulation to orgasm. A 2017 study published in the *Journal of Sex and Marital Therapy* found a wide range in the ways vulva owners orgasm, and in fact, only 18 percent of vulva owners in the study reported experiencing orgasm from penetration alone. This could be because of the variations of nerve endings within the internal vaginal structure, which is why some vulva owners can respond to G-spot (Gräfenberg spot) stimulation alone. The G-spot—better known as the G-area because it differs for everyone and covers an area (not just a spot)—is located inside the vaginal canal on the upper vaginal wall, close to the belly button. So it makes sense that this study would show that most vulva owners need some sort of clitoral stimulation, either on its own or in addition to penetration, to reach climax.

As a 2020 Planned Parenthood article explains: "The clitoris is right under the point where the inner labia meet and form a little hood. It's on top of [or in front of, depending on your angle] the vagina and the urethra [the hole you pee out of]. What you're seeing under that clitoral hood is just the tip of the clitoris." The clitoris is a powerhouse of sexual pleasure, containing approximately eight thousand nerve endings located just in its external anatomy, though it is also composed of a shaft and clitoral legs that straddle the vaginal canal beneath the outer labia (formerly known as the labia majora).

Again in the words of Planned Parenthood: "The clitoris is the pleasure center of the vulva. It doesn't have a central role in reproduction like the penis or vagina, it's pretty much just there to make you feel good!" In other words, when it comes to pleasuring the pussy, the clitoris—and especially its external parts—should be the primary focus for sensation and stimulation.

The Vulva

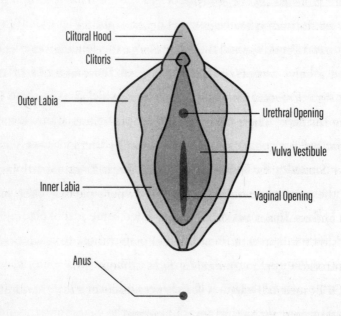

Internal Clitoris

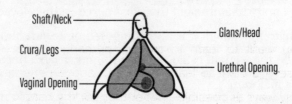

So where did this idea come from that vulva owners should orgasm from penetrative sex alone? And more importantly, why are so many vulva owners (and their partners) continuing to feel outside of the norm when research clearly shows the externally located clitoris is their main resource for pleasure and/or orgasm?

This misinformation has been swirling around since at least the early 1900s. Sigmund Freud viewed the clitoral orgasm as inferior, and he suggested that a vulva owner's inability to orgasm from penetration alone might be a sign of mental illness—a theory later refuted by research from the Kinsey Institute. These false ideas about the clitoris have continued to be debunked for decades in human sexuality textbooks such as the 1980's *Our Sexuality* by Robert Crooks and Karla Baur, identifying the clitoris as the primary resource for a vulva owner's pleasure. Yet, misinformation and confusion persists.

So let's dive in and motorboat the hell out of this juicy question. It's time to introduce you to *Shameless Sex*'s Choose Your Own Pleasure Path (CYOPP) method, which will help you discover the right direction to take on your journey toward sexual freedom.

I HAVE A DIFFICULT TIME ORGASMING

1. Do you want to learn to orgasm primarily to please *yourself—* because you want to learn to orgasm and experience pleasure in as many ways as possible—rather than for the happiness or acceptance of others? If so, continue to read this chapter.

2. Do you want to learn to orgasm in a specific way to please *your partner?* If so, continue to read this chapter. However, we also recommend reading page **170** of **Chapter 5: Are We Broken?** to help

you examine your compatibility with your current partner, as well as page **142** of **Chapter 4: How Can I Ask for What I Want or Even Talk About Sex?** if you feel your underlying issue could benefit from turbocharging your communication skills around sexuality.

3. Are you relating to this sex question as someone struggling with the way your partner orgasms? Do you wish they could orgasm in a certain way? If so, see page **186** of **Chapter 5: Are We Broken?** to contemplate your ability to embrace the way your partner experiences pleasure. Also, continue to read this chapter to gain a better understanding of your partner's perspective.

4. Do you feel like the challenges you are experiencing with orgasm are related to changes in your body, shifts in your mental state, or blocks from past trauma? If so, consider reading on to **Chapter 2: Am I Broken?**

It All Starts with YOU!

Let's talk about self-pleasure, aka masturbation—or as *Shameless Sex* prefers to call it, batin'. You've probably heard some version of the saying "You have to love yourself before someone else can love you." While it may feel daunting or even unattainable to *fully* love yourself, at the very least you can begin to practice more self-love through self-pleasure. That's right, folks—your wanking practice is an important part of mastering the art of self-love and better sex. After all, there is only one person on the planet who can fully understand your body and your pleasure, and that is YOU!

Many people rely on sexual partners to teach them about their own pleasure, but this can lead to confusion and disaster. Unless you're some kind of tried-and-true sexual psychic (and if you are, reach out to *Shameless Sex* because we would love to talk to you), it's not your job to map out someone else's erotic landscape or discern their desires. This is why the number one tool for maximizing your pleasure is all about taking the power back into your own hands (literally).

 Learn more about how to up your batin' game with *Shameless Sex* episodes #224, "Masturbation 101: How to Have GREAT Sex with Yourself—with August McLaughlin," and #282, "Solo Sex and How Batin' Can Lead to Great Sex with Partners—with Mike Mantell."

Whether you're a master at batin' or just starting to investigate the wonders of your body, here are *Shameless Sex*'s top tips to becoming the victor of your vulva, the conqueror of your cock, and the beater of your bits (aka genitals):

Shameless Sex Tips for Uncovering Your O—For you. Yes, YOU!

1. **Practice!** Masturbate often—not just for a couple of minutes a few days here and there, and not by relying on your partner(s) to motivate you. You must create your own self-pleasure practice by making it a regular habit. Start with ten to twenty minutes at least three days a week—and this is key—without making orgasm the objective. You don't have to commit to this forever, but pledging to your pleasure for three to four weeks is recommended. It may feel like work at first,

but the more time you invest into this practice, the easier it becomes. In addition, by dedicating yourself to a regular self-pleasure practice, you are continuously staying connected to your turn-ons and stoking your erotic fire. Once you gain a better understanding for what gets your motor running, you can then share what you've learned with your partner(s), likely resulting in even more pleasure and orgasms.

Put this into action by finding a private place where you will not be interrupted, and put your cell phone on silent (or just turn it off) so you're able to disconnect from the outside world. You can even set the scene by playing your favorite sexy music, lighting some candles, and dressing or undressing yourself so you can drop into your inner sexiness. If the idea of "sexy" doesn't resonate with you, then set a scene that promotes relaxation and safety.

Think of this practice as if you're following a thread of yarn: It's guiding you while you are simultaneously paying attention to each place it wants to take you along the way. Your body's messages are the thread, and if it takes you to your genitals, get after it! If you find that your hands want to rest over your heart or belly, allow that too. No matter where the thread takes you, stay focused on the sensations in the body because you just might find these subtleties to be the stepping stones to a much bigger experience (like orgasm).

2. **Exercise!** You might be thinking, *Wait, what?* But we promise—working on your pelvic floor strength will help you gain control over whatever bits you're rockin'. Have you ever heard of "Kegel exercises"? If not, time to introduce your genitals to pull-ups and presses. It's simple: clench your pelvic floor by pulling it upward toward your body (without hands), hold for two seconds, then release

in a way so it feels like your pelvic floor is moving away from your body. This can feel like you're pushing out or bearing down. Think about what your body does when you have to stop or start urination. Kegel exercises help strengthen your PC (pubococcygeus) muscles, leading to more control over your genitals (including ejaculations for penis owners) and can heighten orgasmic potential. Doing your Kegel exercises for a few minutes a day at least three days a week throughout the year can lead to more powerful orgasms—and even to better bladder control.

3. **Meditate!** Meditation isn't just for yogis and monks. It's a scientifically proven way to reduce the constant chatter inside your mind by steering your attention toward a focal point like your breath or a repeated sound or phrase. Make a commitment to meditate for five to ten minutes a day for at least one week. If you don't know where to begin, try a short, guided meditation available through mindfulness apps or search the internet for the loads of free content specifically designed to help people learn to drop into their bodies. You can also try body scan meditations, where you close your eyes and breathe into different zones of your body from the top of your head down to the tips of your toes.

Once you have the skill down, you can carry these practices over into sex. For most people, deeply connected, pleasurable sex involves a similar single point of focus on the sensations in the body, and training yourself in this focus outside of a sexual context can help you learn to get out of your head. The process might sound abstract, but doing this as a daily habit can help you reconnect with your body, heart, genitals, and breath, and create a sense of acceptance of yourself and others. So, take a deep breath and give yourself permission to try something new—what do you have to lose?

4. **Let go of goals!** Move away from orgasm goals and create awareness around moments when goals get in the way of your presence. If you absolutely have to have a goal, then set it as self-discovery, as you are identifying pleasurable sensation(s) in your body. Since a goal's focus is on the end result, focusing on one can interfere with your ability to stay present for the sensations in your body. So try to make that goal more like an intention to create a deeper connection with yourself instead of a desired future outcome. It's about noticing the subtle sensations along the way. If you want a more specific focus, then take inventory of where you feel sensation—like warmth, tingling, pressure, pleasure, pulsating, pain, numbness, etc.

5. **Fake it till you make it!** No, not your orgasms. When you embark on a self-pleasure session, toss aside any notions that orgasm is unattainable or that you can only feel pleasure in one way. Instead, let your mind work its magic in guiding you towards orgasm and pleasure, by convincing yourself it's within reach and that it can happen—no, that it WILL happen. Barbara Carrellas explains that by taking deeper, fuller breaths and holding positive affirmations in your mind, you may give yourself a higher chance of achieving orgasmic bliss anyway. Similarly, Forrest Andrews, a sex toy designer for Aneros, recommends having a pleasure mantra for experiencing the pleasure you desire—*I'm about to cum, I'm about to orgasm, I'm feeling extreme pleasure. This feels amazing.* This tip has been a game changer for us during many sexy-time sessions—solo as well as with partners.

6. **Consider a porn break!** Or rather, be intentional with your consumption of pornography. While porn can be great for entertainment, it's not realistic. Porn often shows a vulva-owning actor having orgasms from being "pounded out" with little warm up, and most clitoral stimulation is shown via a fast-fondling motion (if there's any fondling of the external bits at all). Porn performers are professionals who are (hopefully) paid to make sex look a certain way—so don't be fooled into believing that sex and orgasm should happen the way they're portrayed on camera.

If you're unsure what kind of stimulation you require for pleasure or orgasm, check out OMGyes (www.omgyes.com/shameless). OMGyes is a platform that demonstrates techniques and shares insights around sexual pleasure via large-scale pleasure-based research studies. OMGyes compiled their research findings into different "seasons" of tasteful video demonstrations and beautiful simulations so folks could bring their learnings into the bedroom. It's an incredible resource, and there's nothing else like it. Though this resource isn't free, using our link will nab you a pretty sweet discount.

Now you may be thinking, *yes yes, Amy and April, I get it, there's nothing wrong with me, and I know how to stimulate myself—but I still want to learn how to orgasm internally.* Well, now that we've covered these *Shameless Sex* tips, we're ready to answer that question. We recommend that you train your body by including internal stimulation in your self-pleasure practice. Start by pleasuring yourself in the way you're typically accustomed to. Then, as you notice yourself getting aroused, and you feel closer to orgasm or have a strong amount of pleasurable sensation in your body, add internal stimulation *while* continuing with the external stimulation. After you feel confident that you can reach orgasm with the two simultaneously, switch it up a bit and remove any external stimulation when you feel yourself getting close to orgasm or deep pleasure. Over time, this technique will help your brain release dopamine and associate pleasure with the internal stimulation, teaching your body to respond more powerfully to it.

It's obvious that vulva owners aren't the only ones feeling alone or different from the rest. There are plenty of penis owners experiencing just as much trauma, hurt, and shame, who also have the same probing question of *Am I normal?* So if you're feeling like you're having orgasms sooner or later than you'd like or as though you don't have control over the hardness of your cock, don't worry, because there are plenty of options out there just for you. It's time to see what you can do with that mighty sex organ sitting between your ears.

I DON'T KNOW HOW TO CONTROL MY PENIS'S PERFORMANCE

My cock does not always perform the way I want it to. Sometimes it goes soft when I am fully turned on. Sometimes I orgasm way before I want to, and I feel like this can't be normal for my age. I should also add that this was a big issue in my last long-term relationship because my girlfriend was continuously unsatisfied with our sex. What should my penis and I do?

Questions around performance issues and the normalcy of the hardness and stamina of the penis seem to be a common concern for penis owners of all ages. People want to know: *Am I hard enough compared to other penis owners? Do I have sex long enough and the way I'm supposed to with my partner? Is this normal, or am I just different from everyone else?*

Remember, if your cock isn't working the way you'd like it to, there is nothing wrong with you. This is incredibly normal and could be linked to a variety of things. Sexual performance could be affected by your emotional or psychological state, unpreventable mental or physical barriers, diabetes, cardiovascular disease, neurological disorders, hormonal imbalances, chronic illnesses, medications, or plenty of other potential health-related events—not to mention the normal results of aging. It would in fact be much more unusual if your body and its sexual capacity *didn't* change at some point during your life. We'll talk more in Chapter 2 about how to adapt to changes and health challenges like these. However, in many cases, the difficulties begin with nonmedical problems like stress and shame—intimately connected with the fear of not being "normal."

You mentioned this being a "big issue" in your last relationship because your partner was unsatisfied with the sex you were having. This probably created shame, which in turn can create performance anxiety. It's important for you (and anyone who feels shame) to remember: *there is nothing wrong with you.* Not meeting someone else's sexual needs does not define who you are as a sexual being. They could have been unskilled in asking for what they wanted, or you two may have been misaligned in your sexual desires at that time. The answer to the problem is never "I'm not good enough." So if you have that kind of mentality, it's time for a reality check: this story is not true!

The recurring limiting beliefs that *I'm not going to stay hard, I'm not going to last long enough,* or *I'm not going to be able to please my partner* can develop into powerful neurological pathways that actually change these beliefs into your new reality. Most penis owners will encounter some form of this issue during their lifetime, so whether you have a penis or you just love a penis, it's imperative to understand that ejaculatory control and penis performance issues are nothing to be ashamed of—just normal parts of life. Having an empathetic understanding of these things while providing a safe, loving space, free of shame and blame when performance issues arise, will help penis owners everywhere gain more confidence and control in the bedroom.

I DON'T KNOW HOW TO CONTROL MY PENIS'S PERFORMANCE

1. Do you want to learn to orgasm primarily to please *yourself*—because you want to learn to harness your ultimate sexual capacity—rather than for the happiness or acceptance of others? If so, continue to read this chapter.

2. Do you want to learn to last longer or stay harder primarily to please *your partner* and satisfy the sexual pleasure they have with you? If so, continue to read this chapter. We also recommend reading **Chapter 7: How Can I Have a Hotter, Steamier, More Connected Sex Life?** for different ways to play no matter what's happening with your body.

3. Do you want to learn more about adapting to the physiological changes in your body? Do you want to find acceptance and tools to work with what you've got? If so, we recommend moving forward to page **83** of **Chapter 2: Am I Broken?**

4. Are you partnered with someone struggling with performance issues or body changes? If so, we recommend reading page **213** of **Chapter 6: How Can I Become a Better Lover?** as a means of learning new ways to both sexually pleasure and support your partner's unique erotic landscape. Also, read page **146** of **Chapter 4: How Can I Ask for What I Want or Even Talk About Sex?** if you're feeling uneasy about approaching a potentially challenging conversation about sex.

It's About Control, Not Dysfunction

Keeley Rankin, MA, sex and relationship coach and an expert in struggling sexual performance in penis owners, prefers using far less limiting terms than "erectile dysfunction" and "premature ejaculation" to describe genital functioning challenges. Instead, she uses the term *erectile and ejaculatory control*. This term emphasizes the point we've been making all along—that despite your frustrations, challenges, or feelings of inadequacy, you are normal and far from alone. Understanding this deep truth is a necessary first step on the journey toward positive change.

> There are several episodes of *Shameless Sex* focused on performance issues, including episodes #184, "Premature Ejaculation, Delayed Ejaculation, and ED— with Keeley Rankin," #208, "Sexual Self-Mastery: Be the Man the World Needs, and the One She Craves—with Destin Gerek," and #231, "Orgasm, Pleasure Challenges & How to Overcome Them—with Dr. Nan Wise."

As Rankin explains, performance challenges are often related to internal anxiety. The story *I'm not going to be able to do the thing I want to do* perpetuates itself, as anxiety and arousal become confusingly intertwined. Rankin suggests, "Think about an imaginary curve that goes from ONE to TEN as arousal builds in the body: ONE is *I'm a little bit interested*, FOUR is *I'm hard enough to penetrate something*, NINE is *I'm at the point of no return and about to orgasm*, and TEN is *I'm having an orgasm*. As the body starts to build arousal the anxiety increases at the same rate." This means that there can be a correlation between arousal and anxiety, in addition to lots of other possible factors affecting penis performance—including those unrelated to internal anxiety. We'll discuss some of those pieces later too.

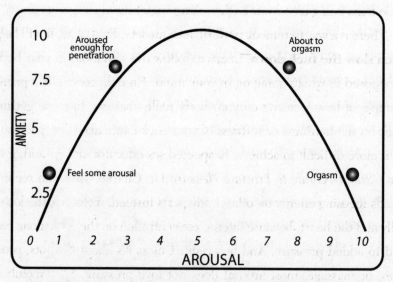

PERFORMANCE CHALLENGE CURVE

Erectile Control

Rankin stresses the direct correlation between erectile control and performance anxiety. She relates it to the old "chicken and egg" scenario. She explains how not getting an erection with a partner at one time could lead to the belief that the same thing will happen the next time as well.

She says the best tool for people who are learning to come back from an erotic shutdown in their bodies around erectile control is to "learn about the sensations and how to follow them in the body. Let the body continue to move toward the sensations without blocking them. Because many times, it's a defense system that causes the performance anxiety, the fear of *Am I going to get hard? Do they like me? Are they going to think my is cock is big enough?*" And instead of facing the possibility of these fears being true, your body—along with your cock—shuts down.

There is a way to remedy performance anxiety. First of all, it will help if you **slow the fuck down**. Learn to follow the sensations in your body as opposed to what's going on in your mind. Erectile control is a prime example of how focusing on your body really matters, because getting stuck on the hardness or softness of your cock can make what you want even more difficult to achieve. Respected sex educator and co-author of *The Ultimate Guide to Prostate Pleasure* Dr. Charlie Glickman recommends focusing energy on other body parts instead, including the lower belly and the heart, because intense concentration on the cock alone can lead to added pressure. And he's right. Unless it's about G-spots, prostates, or massage, most arousal does not love pressure. So remember: pressure does *not* equal pleasure.

The Penis

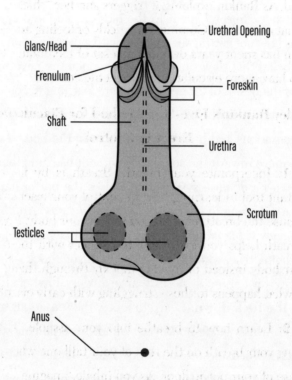

Urethral Opening

Glans/Head

Frenulum

Foreskin

Shaft

Urethra

Scrotum

Testicles

Anus

Ejaculatory Control

When it comes to ejaculatory control, Rankin emphasizes the importance of learning how to maintain arousal. She says, "A lot of people pass over that five on the arousal curve, and the body just shoots over into ejaculation because there's no relationship with how to hold arousal in the body." This problem speaks to a common disconnect between the mind and the body—and specifically, where the mind has taken over. Unfortunately, the more frequent and familiar this experience, the more stressed and stuck you can feel, reinforcing a self-perpetuating combination of anxiety and arousal. As Rankin explains, it triggers another "chicken or egg" situation: "What came first? Coming too quickly or feeling anxious about it?"

Rankin has spent years developing a set of techniques to teach people how to have more ejaculatory and erectile control:

Keeley Rankin's Five-Step Method for Ejaculatory and Erectile Control

Step 1: Incorporate your breath. Breath is by far the most important tool in learning how to control your ejaculation. This is because the breath enables you to feel your body. Focusing on the breath helps you learn how to connect with the sensations in your body instead of moving quickly through them, which is often what happens to those struggling with early ejaculation.

Step 2: Learn how to breathe into your asshole. This means focusing your breath on the root of your tailbone where it meets the base of your pelvic floor. As you inhale, imagine your breath going into your anus. When the body orgasms, your whole pelvic floor pulses and contracts. People who are moving quickly up the arousal curve often start to clench their pelvic floor muscles around the anus in an attempt to stop ejaculation, but this actually tightens those muscles, causing an adverse outcome. Instead, simply breathe into your asshole and release those muscles.

Step 3: Understand how you experience the arousal curve. You can track where you're at on the curve, from one to ten, through your breath. Then begin to separate the arousal curve from the anxiety curve. Oftentimes those two very dissimilar things become one. Can you hang out at five in arousal while letting your anxiety be at two or three?

Step 4: Surf the sweet spot. Focus on a pleasurable sensation in your body, then pinpoint a location within your body where you are experiencing that pleasurable sensation—such as a tingle in your ear, a throbbing in your groin, or the thumping of your heartbeat. Next try to comfortably stay attuned to that sweet place of sensation without letting your anxiety bring you down on the arousal curve. If you find yourself getting too high on the arousal curve, use the anal breathing from Step 2 to bring yourself back down. Repeat as necessary.

Step 5: Learn how to spread the erotic energy over your entire body. Often, there's an overfocus on the sensations of the cock, and you can forget what's happening in the rest of the body, which starts to tense and tighten. Instead, imagine the erotic sensations traveling over your whole body, creating a sense of soft euphoric relaxation so you're able to release, breathe, slow everything down, and start to allow the pleasure to happen.

The best way to become more in tune with your body is to practice self-awareness, says Rankin. "How do you bring everything back to pleasure? You do it by relating to your body again, slowing down, and seeing if you can just enjoy the experience." After all, you can't change a thought pattern you aren't aware of. Notice your sexual cues and pay attention to what you're feeling. By identifying these patterns and recognizing how you think, feel, and act around ejaculatory and erectile control, you can work to challenge them and break their hold over your life. Soon, you may even be able to experience sexual pleasure without orgasm or ejaculation at all.

NORMAL IS UP TO YOU

No matter your situation, getting older inevitably brings about a transformation in how you experience your body. And although sex plays a crucial role in your overall well-being, discussing it with your partner can be intimidating and awkward—especially if you're facing performance issues. However, the more candid you are in expressing your feelings, the better you'll become at understanding your body and identifying what is pleasurable for you. This not only helps you determine if everything's up to snuff when you're feeling like your best self, but also encourages further communication and exploration when something's amiss. While there are a million reasons someone might experience sexual pleasure differently from their partner, it's important to remember that this doesn't make them "less of a person" or "not normal." The only person who can answer this question is you, and what you think and feel is not a reflection of your partner's or anyone else's experience.

Dr. Nagoski sums up normalcy perfectly. She says, "We know by now there's no such thing as normal, or rather, that we're all normal. We are all made of the same parts, they're just organized in different ways. No two alike." So anytime you're doubting your sexual adequacy or ability to fit into societal standards, remind yourself of this: *There is no such thing as normal, and that's a beautiful thing.*

Am I Broken?

For many individuals, the question of *Am I normal?* can get intertwined with *Am I broken?* Believing that they couldn't possibly be normal—and holding the accompanying shame and trauma of this belief—causes concern that something is wrong with who they are as a sexual being. Worries such as *Will I be this way forever? Am I a bad person? Is this feeling ever going to go away?* come up and can linger. However, just as everyone has their own distinct characteristics, which are each themselves "normal," *no one* is broken. We'll say it again: *There is nothing wrong with you!*

Many people particularly struggle with this question when their experience of sexuality takes an unexpected turn—whether it's due to a trauma response, contracting an STI, or physical changes in ability for age- or health-related reasons. In Chapter 1, we shared some perspective on common ways that people see themselves as sexually "abnormal." In this chapter, we'll explore a different aspect of that question: *How do you adapt to sexual changes in your body and mind in a way that brings you closer, rather than further, from your desires?*

The stigma of these changes, and accompanying self-critical beliefs like those around so-called "brokenness," can be traumatic. *Shameless Sex* **does not** believe humans are broken or that people are "damaged goods." We empathize with how hard it is to live with shame and trauma, and we know it may not be fully healable or gone forever, but it *is* workable . . . and that's worth exploring.

THE IMPACT OF SHAME AND TRAUMA ON SEXUALITY

In his book *In the Realm of Hungry Ghosts*, trauma and addiction expert Dr. Gabor Maté emphasizes the impact your past wounding has on your current state of being. This means neglect, trauma, and emotional loss continue far beyond the pain of the traumatic event itself, creating long-term distortions in how you relate to the world. And trauma can stem from a wide variety of things. Even if you don't think your experience was "that bad" (whatever that means), it's important to recognize that there is no hierarchy of trauma. Everyone's experience is subjective, and *all* shame or trauma is valid. However, it's widely understood that some demographics do experience higher rates of trauma. *Shameless Sex* especially acknowledges those humans, as well as anyone lacking the resources to access the tools to heal themselves; we hold immense optimism for a better future where such circumstances no longer exist.

Shame and trauma can happen at any point in your life, yet research shows people are most impressionable during the developmental years of childhood. This means every experience you have from infancy to high school impacts who you are in adulthood. From how you were raised by your parents, to how peers treated you, to any experiences of violence or discrimination, to health problems and natural disasters and your ability to access resources for survival in the physical environment you lived in—the list goes on and on. In fact, a 2017 study published in the journal *Infancy* suggests that external stressors could begin to shape people's lives as early as in utero. The birthing parent's history with trauma as well as additional stressors occurring during pregnancy can impact the child's developmental outcome.

A 2018 UCLA study reinforced this concept. Researchers discovered that childhood adversity and trauma extend across generations, and parents with severe trauma and stresses in childhood were four times more likely to have children with mental health and behavioral problems of their own. In other words, children absorb and personify their parents' perceptions of themselves and are deeply affected by their surroundings in a way that will likely continue into adulthood.

In his groundbreaking book *The Body Keeps the Score*, trauma researcher Bessel van der Kolk, MD, demonstrates how much of an impact trauma has on the mind and body. Dr. van der Kolk's work shows how harrowing experiences can affect the neuroplasticity of the brain, especially in the areas dedicated to pleasure, engagement, control, and trust. Traumatic stress correlates with greater hyperactive arousal in the brain, leading to the release of stress hormones and impaired functioning, often resulting in a highly agitated or panicked state. Conversely, this research also reveals the benefits of neuroplasticity, and how practices such as therapy, breath work, meditation, movement practices, guided medicinal sessions, and even new positive experiences with the self, friends, family, and lovers can help rewire the brain to heal from its experiences of trauma. Though the old neural pathways of trauma won't just go away, working with these new, positive pathways may lead them to become far more powerful than the old pathways of pain were. This means it's possible to transform the damaging, painful story of *I am broken* to something that better serves you and your life now—no matter what was in the past.

Trauma can also be deeply connected to shame. Pioneering shame and vulnerability researcher Brené Brown explains the tipping point between guilt and shame. While guilt—the feeling of "that thing I did is bad"—may serve as a precursor for shame, many people move through it over time. On the other hand, shame—the feeling that "I am bad" or "I am broken"—can act like a parasite, penetrating every cell of yourself, paralyzing you with limiting beliefs about who you are. A lot of people deal with this by burying shame and trauma deep within the shadows of themselves as a protective mechanism. But these tactics are only a temporary fix. As Brown's work suggests, silence and secrecy tend to intensify shame, and those protective walls will get in the way of connection as well as shame's antidote: empathy. You can't just stick a shame Band-Aid on things and expect to be able to move on.

To put it bluntly, most people have some sort of unresolved trauma or shame inside of them. They won't always be able to identify the source, either—maybe it didn't seem to be impactful at the time (or maybe it wasn't their trauma at all!) and only emerged later as a significant factor in their life. Identifying and working to shift any unresolved shame or trauma is a crucial initial step toward having optimal sexual experiences.

I WANT TO ENJOY SEX AFTER EXPERIENCING TRAUMA

I have never orgasmed in my life—even with a sex toy. I experienced a fair amount of sexual trauma when I was younger and have felt a lot of shame about it. I didn't start masturbating until my first year of college, even though I started having sex in high school. At the time, I barely understood consent or that my pleasure mattered, and I continue to struggle with this. I see a therapist and am trying to work through my trauma, and even though I can get close to having an orgasm, I feel like there's a block that has never let me cross the threshold. Is there a way I can work through this or am I totally broken?

The first step when you are navigating through past trauma is to seek support in a safe space with a trusted professional. While it's usually helpful to have awareness of the wounds from the past, depending on the degree of trauma and how your mind and body react when trauma enters your psyche, this cognizance may cause more emotional harm if the uncovering process is done alone, which is why working with a therapist and/or a well-trained professional is imperative as you revisit the past.

As of 2022, current statistics from the National Sexual Violence Resource Center indicate around 81 percent of vulva owners and 43 percent of penis owners report experiencing some form of sexual harassment or assault in their lifetime. So remember that you are not alone.

On a positive note, it *is* possible to have fulfilling sexual experiences after trauma. Dr. Nan Wise, certified sex therapist, cognitive neuroscientist, and author of *Why Good Sex Matters*, elaborates on the process of recovery: "The work [involves] a different know-how, discharging the emotions that are associated with these painful experiences, and ultimately letting the person go to a place where they focus their attention on harnessing the sensations of the experience so they can allow their orgasm to find them. And the orgasm will."

 Dr. Nan shares her life's work in understanding sexual pleasure, including challenges with orgasm, in episode #231, "Orgasm, Pleasure Challenges, and How To Overcome Them—with Dr. Nan Wise."

Both Amy and April have personally discovered the power of going beyond standard talk therapy by exploring other holistic methodologies with experienced practitioners who provide a safe space for you to heal. These methods, including EMDR (eye movement desensitization and reprocessing) therapy, hypnotherapy, Somatic Experiencing, and inner child work, can each offer profound results for the mind, body, and spirit.

No matter which therapeutic approaches you decide to pursue, your personal journey is entirely in your hands. You have the choice to pick the Pleasure Path that your unique system needs to facilitate the healing process. And remember, while you undertake this journey, it's essential to be compassionate towards yourself every step of the way.

I WANT TO ENJOY SEX AFTER EXPERIENCING TRAUMA

1. Do you want to work on this blockage with a professional who specializes in something other than talk therapy for current shame or past trauma? If so, continue to read this chapter.

2. Do you want to learn some tools to help you orgasm on your own? If so, continue to read this chapter.

3. Do you want to learn how to find the right sex toy to use in a way that works for your body? If so, go to page **116** of **Chapter 3: How Do I Know What I Want in the Bedroom?** for sex toy recommendations and various ways to implement them into your life.

Get ready to bust a move or do a little happy dance because you are on the verge of uncovering significant opportunities for growth. Whether you want to work with someone who can support your quest to go deeper into your body to learn about the shame and trauma it holds or you're looking for tools to apply on your own time, know that (though it can be a little dark and stormy at times) your future is bright, so you better find some shades.

Finding the Right Therapist or Coach Matters

If you're interested in working through trauma or shame with professionals, we have a few tips we'd like to share. First of all, current research emphasizes the importance of moving beyond talk therapy by also exploring the experiences the body undergoes when feeling challenged or triggered—so if you're sensing your therapeutic container (the energy you feel via the one-on-one engagement with your therapist) is targeting your mind but not simultaneously engaging your body's present experiences, you may want to consider a different container. This could entail asking your current therapist to help navigate your internal somatic space or, if they are unable to do so, take Dr. Nan's advice and find a therapist who can.

Dr. Nan suggests, "The old methods of working with trauma [by] just talking about it are not really that helpful. It's the releasing of emotions that can be incredibly transformational . . . All of that self-consciousness you're experiencing is a symptom of anxiety. And anxiety, I know very well since I'm a long-term anxiety sufferer. The tools you need to work with are the body, the breath, and the mind because they all can help you relax into experiencing sexual pleasure."

LMFT and sex therapist Melissa Fritchle advises those seeking a new therapist, support person, or coach that "whoever [this person] is, ideally is going to help you find a balance where you're touching on the pain and you're able to address it. But you're also simultaneously having the sense that 'I'm safe in this moment' where you can look at this pain and be received, accept yourself, breathe, and not feel completely overwhelmed in the moment." At this point, you may be thinking: *This seems like a lot to ask for from my therapist.* And in certain circumstances, you may be right. In fact, many people have multiple coaches and therapists, each trained to focus on specific areas of challenge and necessity. **Pro Tip**: Inform your different practitioners about each other—this helps prevent any conflict of interest that may arise.

 Let these experts further guide you in finding your dream therapist(s) and the right professionals for you in episodes #141, "Healing Sexual Trauma Through Pleasure—with Melissa Fritchle, LMFT," and #268, "How to Find the Right (Sex and Relationship) Therapist or Coach—with Keeley Rankin, MA."

Dr. Nan Wise and Melissa Fritchle both have years of practice in the field of sexuality and agree on the importance of working with someone trained to help you venture into this profound part of the inner psyche. As time goes on, society is becoming more aware of the importance of body-centric therapeutic modalities. There were a few previously mentioned on page 62, but if you'd like some additional options, we can recommend the Hakomi Method, IFS (Internal Family Systems), and Sexological Bodywork to name just a few. Always be sure any practitioner you seek is well-trained and qualified.

Tools for Working Through Your Sexual Barriers

Below are some gentle steps, courtesy of the knowledgeable Melissa Fritchle, so you can dip a toe in and test the waters before jumping into the deep end of working through your sexual barriers.

1. **Presence**: If it's a challenge to come into presence—the process of slowing down—it's helpful to stay open to all the ways you can feel your body (joy, pleasure, sensation, etc.). A lot of people get set on sex being one way: there's orgasm and extreme pleasure, or the body is turned off and numb or even in pain. But with presence comes these little in-between experiences of subtle sensation . . . a little tingling, a little warmth, a little pulsating, and so on.

   For a lot of people with traumatic memories, sitting in your own mind is often not comfortable, which can make mindfulness difficult. Yet you can still be mindful of the body and its sensations—feel your own touch on your skin, drop into a sensation you like, or focus on a taste you enjoy. Take time to discover the more subtle sensations on your own, as it's easier to be mindful and aware when it's just you in the room.

2. **Connect with your body**: Learn to say, "My body is an ally and an okay place to be," especially if your heart and body feel conflicted (for example, "My heart wants to have sex, but my body reacts as though I don't"). This may feel like your body is lying, but that's not the case; your body is asking you to go a little slower. Your body is being hyperaware, hyperalert, and making sure things are okay. It also doesn't mean you can't trust your heart and your mind. You could be thinking *I want to be sexual right now*, but if your body is responding with fear, that's a sign for you to reassure your body: *We might need to slow down right now*. Make sure you're checking in with what helps you feel safe and secure, and that you can communicate your needs. Think of it as a new way to establish a deeper connection with your body.

3. **Use your senses**: Not sure where to start? During solo sexual exploration, consider the following questions: *What's the softest place on my body?* Find that zone. *What's the warmest place right now?* Explore that area. Utilize all five senses to focus on what can bring you into little bouts of pleasure. Concentrate on being in the present moment with your body. That will lead to better sexual sensation, and any awakening of sensation can contribute to a deeper understanding of your body along with more enjoyment of that experience.

4. **Create awareness**: It's possible that certain areas of your body are not yet ready for intense sensation. Notice and acknowledge these parts and treat them gently. In situations like this, there are little ways to create self-awareness and recognize that you have the ability to feel even the most subtle of sensations. In time, you may discover that your body is ready and eager to engage with you and provide you with pleasure.

Addressing Pain and Reframing Shame

If negative experiences with your body have impacted you in ways you prefer to ignore, engaging in a dialogue with your body, specifically your genitals, can be helpful. Recognize the ways you've disregarded your body's messages, and then commit to do better and be gentle with yourself. This process is about identifying the hurt that happened in the past, as well as how you've treated your body to cope with and endure that hurt.

For an example of this practice, you could place one hand over your heart or belly while the other is cupping your genitals, then take a deep breath and say something like, "I am deeply sorry for all the ways I did not listen to you. I know you never asked for this, yet I still don't listen to you. I vow to do my best to show up for you in a better way. I want to honor you and all of me." If this seems ridiculous, just know that it has been transformational for Amy in her path toward better emotional and sexual self-care. Taking the time to acknowledge and speak to these parts of yourself allows you to interrupt any disconnection with your body and potentially bring yourself "online" again, so your body, mind, and genitals are working together as one.

To take this "conversation" a step further, Somatica practitioner and certified sexological bodyworker Dolly Josette suggests mastering the language of your body. With a gentle single-point touch, you can "map" your genitals, bringing awareness, focus, and intention to the physical and emotional sensations of your body. This approach can aid in honing the skill of listening to the body's signals, thus fostering trust and acceptance between you and your body.

If shame comes up around self-pleasuring, consider reframing the experience altogether. Sex educator, pleasure products developer, and repeat *Shameless Sex* guest Kristen Tribby suggests asking yourself a couple of questions like *How can you make your shame sexy?* and *How can you invite the erotic into your fantasies as a means of working with the hurt, disconnect, or pain?* Your reframing process will be distinctive to you.

For example, you might reclaim your power over past shame or trauma by incorporating it into your sex life with a kinky twist—where you're choosing what's happening and you have control over the circumstances. This approach could even lead you to a new source of arousal. You could also have a masturbation session where you fantasize about feeling deeply seen and cared for by someone you visualize.

You might also consider the ingenious strategy recommended by sexual visionary Layla Martin. Imagine a crowd cheering for you during your self-pleasure session. Embrace this, and try to find a way to make it playful, fun, or pleasurable. Design your make-believe spectators and their actions however you like. Maybe they're hollering, "Fuck yes! Get after it! You deserve all the pleasure in the world!" or, "Watching you touch yourself is so hot, it makes us all want to touch ourselves too," or maybe they're just doing a synchronized wave and fist pumping in unison. The choice is entirely up to you.

These educators' suggestions for moving through shame and trauma around sexuality are closely aligned with what *Shameless Sex* stands for. As we described in "The *Shameless Sex* Philosophy," some of the most valuable tools in your erotic tool kit involve focusing on *you* and slowing down in almost all aspects of sexuality. That's why it's vital to take the time to learn about your body and its unique expression of arousal and desire. In other words, don't expect someone else to teach you about your own pleasure; it's your fundamental right and it's your body, so take the time to understand it.

There is no doubt the tools above are most impactful when applied alongside a strong and experienced support system. But even without this, forward movement is possible when you take small, slow steps toward shifting your own behavioral practices or ways of thinking. If this seems confusing, remember—go slower than slow, then slower than that!

 Expand your knowledge of ways to both heal and eroticize your trauma with episodes #142, "Cum Fetishes, Lingerie Fetishes, Virginity, and More—with Kristen Tribby," and #102, "Awakening the Yoni: Vulva Mapping—with Sexological Bodyworker Dolly Josette."

I'M LIVING WITH AN STI/STD AND DON'T FEEL SEXUALLY CONFIDENT

I was diagnosed with genital herpes three years ago, but I've never had symptoms. Can I actually have herpes or an STD without ever showing symptoms? Is this something I need to warn partners about, and what if they reject me? Is this the end of my sexy single life?

To all humans who have been diagnosed with an STI (sexually transmitted infection, formerly known by the less-accurate term STD, or sexually transmitted disease): You are not alone! When April was diagnosed with genital herpes in her late teens, at first she encountered shame and manipulation from those she shared her diagnosis with—leading to years of self-deprecating feelings, loneliness, and relationship stagnation. Amy has also been diagnosed with STIs at varying stages of her life, such as HSV-1 (herpes simplex virus/oral cold sores) from an innocent make-out session at age eighteen as well as HPV (human papillomavirus) years into a monogamous relationship at age twenty-one—followed by chlamydia not once but *twice* in her late twenties from encounters involving "just the tip" of the penis (aka JTT).

STIs Happen

If you're thinking Amy and April are just two irresponsible humans who should have been more careful, then it's past time to get that out of your system. Go ahead, Judge Judy, knock yourself out and shame the *Shameless Sex* duo. But if you're ready for a reality check, it might be time to put down your gavel because guess what? STIs happen and are very common! And while you're at it, ponder this: Your judgment is likely just a reflection of everything you've been told is dirty and wrong with people who have sex with multiple partners—or with sex in general. This could even be a reflection of how you feel about your own perceived flaws, or of your shame, trauma, and insecurities about sex and relationships.

Regardless of their trigger, if feelings of judgment or discomfort arise, let yourself feel them. Then, take a breath and check in with yourself. Identify with those feelings and try your best to move through them. Also, consider the notion that if you're a human having sex in the twenty-first century, *STIs can happen*. Simply put, if you have sex with another person, you could contract an STI, and there is a chance you could transmit it to another partner—even when you're being "careful" and applying safer sex practices.

What Is "Safer Sex"?

"Safer sex" refers to anything people do to lower their risk, and their partners' risk, of sexually transmitted infections. Some call it "safe sex," but since no type of sex with a partner can be guaranteed to be completely safe, this is not quite accurate. For this reason, think of sexual safety behaviors as existing on a spectrum. On one side of the spectrum, there is abstinence or nonsexual touch, and as you move toward the other side, you see different actions involving the exchange of body fluids via hands, mouth, genitals, and sex toys—or generally any object or body part that could transmit one person's body fluids to another. As Amy's

Sexually Transmitted Infections
SPECTRUM OF RISK

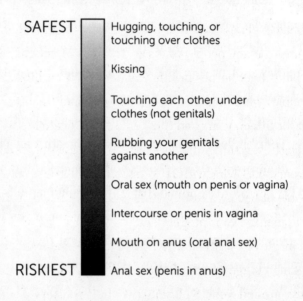

SAFEST

Hugging, touching, or touching over clothes

Kissing

Touching each other under clothes (not genitals)

Rubbing your genitals against another

Oral sex (mouth on penis or vagina)

Intercourse or penis in vagina

Mouth on anus (oral anal sex)

RISKIEST

Anal sex (penis in anus)

two JTT infections reflect, it doesn't take full-on penetration for infections, diseases, and bacteria to be shared.

The more sexually active humans that are living, fucking, making love, JTTing, or even making out in the twenty-first century, the greater the likelihood of contracting some sort of STI. In 2018, the Centers for Disease Control and Prevention reported roughly 48 percent of the US population aged 14–49 had HSV-1 and around 12 percent had HSV-2. The number is even greater with HPV, which approximately 80-plus percent of sexually active people will contract in their lifetime. Despite how widespread STIs are, society continues to view them as the end of the world and some sort of sexual death sentence. Semi-innocent seventeen-year-old April experienced this firsthand—she was literally told by her most trusted peers that her life was over after contracting HSV-1 from her first PIV partner.

Herpes gets an especially bad rap. In the words of pelvic health and intimate wellness expert and *Shameless Sex* guest Remy Paille, NP, "There are so many people who say, 'It's fine if I get chlamydia or gonorrhea, but if I get herpes my life will be over.' Your life is not over . . . I know couples where one of them has herpes and the other one has not gotten it for fifteen years and they're just fine. There are ways to control and mitigate everything. It comes back to the basics of taking really good care of yourself." Living with HSV and other STIs does not make you any less capable of having a fulfilling life as a sexual being. There are plenty of ways to manage your prognosis.

The magic of twenty-first century medicine means there are options when taking charge of your sexual health, but no matter what, having awareness around your STI status is the first step. The second step requires some education around managing how an STI affects your body. While chlamydia and gonorrhea can be cured with a few pills, HSV-1 and HSV-2 remain in your body, although they can be managed well with medications, dietary protocols, as well as an understanding of the shifts that occur within your body. For many people, HSV and other STIs only make a guest appearance every so often (with and without warning), after which the virus goes dormant for months, years, or sometimes a lifetime.

As Paille explains, HPV, for example, "is kind of like having a cold in your genitals that you're probably going to clear eventually, but it might hang out for a few years. If it does, we just keep testing it." Whether you have HPV, a different STI, or none at all, getting routine STI testing can help you responsibly navigate your sexual health, and the process isn't as scary as it seems.

 Get even more informed about STIs in episodes #120, "The STD (aka STI) Episode—with Remy Paille, NP," and #332, "Another STD (aka STI) Episode—with Danielle Bezalel, MPH."

Whether you or your partner(s) are currently living with an STI and know it or you're simply a human living on planet Earth who has considered the probability of getting or giving an STI at some point in your life, there are several Pleasure Paths available to steer you in the right direction.

I'M LIVING WITH AN STI/STD AND DON'T FEEL SEXUALLY CONFIDENT

1. Do you want to not only come to terms with your STI status, but find acceptance and confidence around this matter? If so, continue to read this chapter.

2. Do you want to understand general STI protocol and learn how to ethically navigate this tricky terrain? If so, continue to read this chapter.

3. Do you want to learn how to share STI status and be able to have safer-sex conversations with current or future partner(s)? If so, continue to read this chapter. We also recommend reading page **149** of **Chapter 4: How Can I Ask for What I Want or Even Talk About Sex?** so you can learn how to have difficult conversations around sex.

Modern-Day Medicine and Managing Herpes

First of all—if, like the podcast listener who asked this question you were diagnosed with herpes without ever presenting symptoms, there is a high probability that you're one of the lucky humans whose body sends HSV into a longstanding internal hibernation as opposed to having recurring outbreaks. Many people living with some form of HSV have *never* had symptoms. Additionally, many people can have one or a few outbreaks after which the virus goes dormant in their bodies for long periods of time.

Neither of these are markers of an inability to transmit the virus to others, though, because even folks living with dormant HSV can pass it on. However, in the words of Remy Paille, NP, "theoretically, the likelihood of passing it to a partner is very low, especially when someone hasn't had an outbreak in a long time, is healthy, and not immunocompromised . . . [But] you never know when you're shedding the virus." Because of this, it's important to always be open about your STI diagnoses and we'll discuss how best to do that later in the chapter.

If you *are* having recurring outbreaks, genitally or orally, there are medications available that can be taken daily or as needed and can decrease the likelihood and length of outbreaks. Your diet can also help. Monitoring your intake of arginine, an amino acid, and eating foods rich in lysine, another amino acid, can help. High levels of arginine are found in foods such as oats, nuts, seeds, chocolate, and wheat, and avoiding these foods can reduce outbreak reoccurrences. A high-lysine diet encompasses protein-rich foods like meat, poultry, fish, dairy, and many fruits and vegetables, and eating these foods can help prevent outbreaks from happening. Amy implements a specific diet for two to four days the moment she feels an indication that a cold sore is coming on. She will eat apples, avocados, apricots, figs, beets, and a plethora of vegetables, along with various meats and cheeses. For her, combining this diet with antiviral pills from her doctor, along with (what might be) the most important preliminary step—the awareness of changes in her body—allows her to immediately halt the onset of a long and painful HSV outbreak.

There are specific sensations that occur in the body before and during an outbreak, and when you can learn to recognize these changes, like Amy has, you will be able to take charge of the situation and minimize the virus's impact. The beginning of a herpes outbreak is usually accompanied by a tingling, buzzing, burning, and/or itching sensation in a targeted area of your body. This generally happens in mucous membranes such as the mouth, lips, genitals, or anus, or even other areas of the body (usually those that are warm and moist). You might also experience flu-like symptoms and have a fever, headache, and swollen lymph nodes. Paying attention to bodily shifts like these can help you learn to manage HSV before you start presenting symptoms.

Beyond herpes-specific shifts, though, it also pays to be cautious when you feel stressed or under the weather. Herpes, along with many other recurring STIs, looks at these factors as the perfect opportunity to come in for a visit. During such times, go on a high-lysine diet, consult with your doctor for a prescription (or have one on hand so you're prepared), get ample amounts of sleep, and focus on caring for yourself. If sex is on the table, it's imperative to share where you're at with your current partner(s) so they can choose to abstain from sexual activity until your system rebalances itself.

Possessing a broader understanding of STIs can give you the wherewithal to help navigate future sexual situations. With each occurrence

Reid Mihalko's
SAFER-SEX ELEVATOR SPEECH

**PAUSE for PRESENCE,
POWER DYNAMICS, & PERMISSION**
—Take a breath. Can those involved say yes/no freely?
If yes, seek permission to share . . .

LAST TIME TESTED
—Share when you were last tested, what you were tested for,
and the results of those tests. Congrats! The scariest part is
out of the way!

ESSENTIALS ABOUT ME
—Share whatever "Here's how to win with me" info you want
them to know! *e.g., Pronouns, words not to use, relationship
agreements, etc.*

ADDRESS YOUR SAFER-SEX NEEDS
—Share your safer-sex protocols, safewords, & whatever needs
you have to help address your emotional, spiritual, and
physical health.

SINCE MY LAST TEST
—Share any updates regarding sexual mishaps/risky behavior
(Condom slipped off? Missed birth control? etc.) that could
affect future STI results or other aspects of sexual activity.

USUALLY LIKE
—Share one or two things that you know you usually enjoy
(sexually or non-sexually). Sharing these things doesn't mean
it has to happen.

RATHER NOT
—Share at least one thing you know you don't enjoy
sexually or activities or body parts that are off the menu
for today.

ENQUIRE
—Invite them to share by asking, "And how about you?"

and open discussion of outbreaks, your ability to manage them and comfortably discuss your STI status with others will get easier. You'll gain more confidence and compassion for yourself in the process as well.

How to Shamelessly Share Your STI Status

When it comes to having safer-sex conversations including STI status, we love sex educator Reid Mihalko's "Safer-Sex Elevator Speech" protocol.

Let's go a little more in depth.

- **P is for PAUSE for PRESENCE, POWER DYNAMICS, & PERMISSION.** Before you initiate a safer-sex talk, pause and ask yourself, "Am I clear and present enough to make aligned choices and notice subtle communications from others at this moment?" Take a deep breath. Get grounded. Then consider if there are altered states or individual power dynamics involved that might make it tricky for the other person to say *yes* or *no* clearly and freely. If you're grounded and they are free to say *yes* or *no*, then ask for their permission and their consent to proceed. "Would you be willing to have a safer-sex conversation with me?" If they say no, thank them for taking care of themselves. If they say yes, proceed to the next step.
- **L is for LAST TIME TESTED.** When were you last tested for STIs, what did you get tested for, and what were the results? Share the scariest things first and get them out of the way. This makes the rest of the conversation easier. Plus, you're modeling for the other person that it's not shameful to talk about STIs. If you have tested positive for herpes, HPV, or another long-lasting STI in the past, mention that here.

- **E is for ESSENTIALS ABOUT ME.** Share your "here's how to win with me" info and other important details that will give others a heads-up on how to create a positive experience with you and avoid disastrous assumptions. Are you in an altered or distressed state at the moment? What is your current relationship status and sexual orientation? What, if any, relationship agreements do you have that they should know about? What pronouns do you use? Any dirty talk words they should use or avoid? Are there particular words you like to use for your body parts? Words not to use? What are your expectations? What are your body's needs for comfort? Any injuries or conditions you'd like to share? This is the perfect time to inform people about you.

- **A is for ADDRESS YOUR SAFER-SEX NEEDS.** Share your safer-sex protocols and needs. What emotional, spiritual, and physical health and safety needs do you have? What barriers do you require for certain types of activities? Are you on birth control? If so, what kind(s)? Have you had a vasectomy? What are your protocols and needs if there is a barrier or contraceptive failure resulting in an unwanted pregnancy or a future positive STI test? Do you have other partners whose sexual practices might be relevant to share? Are there ways that you like to negotiate kink and power dynamics? Any potential triggers you might have and safe words they should know about? Ways you like to communicate nonverbally? What about your aftercare/post-sex needs? What are your protocols for handling miscommunications, mishaps, and repairing hurts or triggers? These are big topics, but they get easier the more you practice talking about them.

- **S is for SINCE MY LAST TEST.** Any updates since you were last tested? Have any risky sexual activities or mishaps gone down since your last test? Did a condom break or slip off? Recently forgot to take your birth control? Had recent news that a lover tested positive for something? If so, add this to your safer-sex elevator speech with partners.

- **U is for USUALLY LIKE.** Share one or two things that you know you usually enjoy (sexually or nonsexually). This may or may not be something you want to do with this person. Sharing it doesn't mean it has to happen.

- **R is for RATHER NOT.** Share at least one thing you know you *do not* enjoy sexually, or activities or body parts that are off the menu for you today. Expressing what you're not into is a great way to create trust and show that you know your limits and have words for them. You're also modeling that the other person is allowed to have limits too.

- **E is for ENQUIRE.** The last step is asking, "And how about you?" This is where you invite the other person to share *their* safer-sex talk. Congratulations! Not only did you model for others a great approach to sharing sexual health information and needs, you also have a powerful opportunity to assess where they are in their journey of sexual agency and to learn more about their approach to sexual health and ability to use their words.

This type of conversation is not only helpful for being forthright about safer sex, including current and past STI status, but also helps people deepen their connection. Let's imagine a world where these types of exchanges are the standard, and checking in with future lovers about STI status—while negotiating each person's wants and needs to navigate safer sex together—is the norm. In this world, everyone feels heard, and consent reigns over all with pleasure right by its side. Well, guess what? This doesn't have to be imaginary. By having these conversations, you can make it happen—leading everyone to have even hotter (safer) sex.

Having these interactions enables everyone involved to access informed consent and feel as safe and comfortable as possible in their bodies and sexualities. In the words of Remy Paille, "Oftentimes it's just the thought of having the conversation that's uncomfortable, but when you start having it, it can actually feel good . . . Just ask yourself, 'Now that I know this person's been truly honest with me, then what happens if I do get an STI?' or 'What happens if I have unprotected sex and I get pregnant?' Have a plan so you can calm your anxiety. 'What if I get an STI? Then what? I'll go get treated. Then what? I'll have to call everybody I've slept with recently and tell them. Then what? Then they'll have to call everybody they've slept with. Then we're all going to get tested. Then we're all going to get treated.' Make your decision from that vantage point." In this way, safer-sex conversations also prepare you to respond quickly, responsibly, and with less stress. And, as Paille emphasizes, "It's crucial to give and get informed consent about STI results because from there you can consent if you want to go further—knowing [the risks] and understanding how you're going to treat it if you do end up with the same thing."

Engaging in these types of difficult conversations can allow you to develop a deep sense of security as you validate the significance of your own needs and receive your sexual partner's full acceptance and honesty regarding their own needs. Together, you're building a place where mind, body, and genitals all feel a big YES to the circumstances at hand.

Other Common Infections

What about other common infections like candida (yeast infection) and BV (bacterial vaginosis, caused by excessive growth of vaginal bacteria and not technically an STI)? If you're experiencing symptoms like itching, unusual discharge, or something else that's out of the ordinary, your doctor can perform tests to figure out the problem and the appropriate treatment.

For BV and candida, Paille recommends boric acid suppositories as treatment, which help restore vaginal flora to its optimal state, encouraging the growth of good bacteria and discouraging the growth of bad bacteria. She explains, "The vaginal microbiome can get thrown off from the tip of the penis, semen, or just something that you had a reaction to. Then other bacteria that live in your vaginal canal, like [Gardnerella,] the one that causes BV, grows, and when too much is present, the vaginal pH gets thrown off. Then the Gardnerella bacteria has little bacteria bug babies, and they grow and proliferate. It all starts with one bacteria bug, which is why it's not going to show up on a test until all the bugs have had babies and there's a colonization. A lot of [vulva owners] get BV and have it for a long time not understanding what it is—they just know that something feels off or smells different in their vaginas."

I'M ON MEDICATION AND IT'S AFFECTED MY SEXUAL PLEASURE

I don't have a problem getting an erection, but I can't seem to reach orgasm, even with masturbation. I am on several medications that help with my mental well-being and depression. Is this just who I am now? If not, what are ways I can remedy this?

We've received a wide array of emails from people of all genders regarding how prescription medications affect pleasure and sexual function. The side effects of many medications can, indeed, impact a person's sexuality, regardless of their age or level of health in other areas.

Cha-Cha-Changes and Aging

All humans inevitably change as they age. Just think about it—close your eyes and imagine a sixty-year-old person. Think about the work their (or your) body has done over the years to keep that person alive. Really think about all the systems at play: the skin protecting, the lungs breathing, the heart pumping, the stomach digesting, the blood circulating—and that's just a few of this body's basic functions. You can think of the body like a car; the more miles it's driven, the more parts need to be replaced, tires changed, and fluids topped off, even with proper tune-ups and regular trips to the mechanic. Similarly, the human body—even with proper tune-ups—will function differently with each orbit around the sun.

All you need is an openness to work with what is present while considering the shifts at hand. And this applies to penises, vulvas (not to be confused with "Volvos"; we obviously love a car comparison, but we're done for now), and other bits, because all genitals and their sexual function will change with age. This encompasses everything including elasticity, lubrication, orgasms, and libido.

 Keep things hot at any age with episodes #127, "How to Have Hot Sex at Any Age—with Joan Price," and #131, "Boners and ED—with Dr. John Carrozzella."

Cha-Cha-Changes and Life's Curveballs

Sometimes change comes from unexpected occurrences that result in chronic pain, disability, and other challenging circumstances. Genetic diseases, compromising conditions resulting in loss of sensation or function in areas of the body, prenatal and birth complications, and other medical difficulties can all have a major impact on sex and relationships—especially when folks with the above experiences feel pressure to fit into the über-shiny standard of what is "normal." As emphasized in Chapter 1, abnormal is the real normal, and as long as you are abiding by consent, there is no wrong way to be a sexual human being.

A lot of people suffer from the false belief that they are broken. It's also a shitty reality to exist in. We empathize with these feelings, and indeed part of this book's goal is to provide options to anyone who reads it, including those facing life-altering events that have led to an unsatisfying sex life. If this is you, we want you to know that pleasure and sexual connection are still available to you, regardless of the curveballs life throws your way. So put on your catcher's mitt (and mask too—safety first, everyone) because it's time to find the pitch that works as you CYOPP and slide into whatever base feels like home.

I'M ON MEDICATION AND IT'S AFFECTED MY SEXUAL PLEASURE

1. Are you curious about how to talk to your doctor about your sexual challenges in hopes of finding a balance between the medications you require and the sexual pleasure you crave? If so, continue to read this chapter.

2. Do you want to learn how to have orgasms or experience fulfilling pleasure regardless of the medications you're taking? If so, read this chapter. We also recommend going back to page **49** of **Chapter 1: Am I Normal?** to get a better understanding of control versus dysfunction.

3. Do you want to experience sex and pleasure in new ways that take into account the shifts in your body? If so, continue to read this chapter. We also recommend going back to page **46** of **Chapter 1: Am I Normal?** to gain a better understanding of the shifts that can happen in your body.

4. Is your ultimate desire to create more acceptance with your body's changes and learn how to work with what is present for you now? If so, go to page **264** of **Chapter 7: How Can I Have a Hotter, Steamier, More Connected Sex Life?**

Medication and Sex

Before getting to this question about "delayed ejaculation"—a process that can occur for penis owners of all ages for various reasons—let's first hone in on prescription medications, especially those for mental health treatment, and how they can affect sexuality.

First and foremost, while medications like selective serotonin reuptake inhibitors (SSRIs, a common type of antidepressant) are not a "perfect" solution, the mental and emotional improvements they may cause in people who struggle with mental illness are incredibly significant. However, according to sex therapist Melissa Fritchle, "around 75 percent of people who take SSRIs experience sexual side effects [including] lower libido, as well as erectile or orgasmic difficulties, and painful ejaculation. Duration and intensity of orgasm changes dramatically for people as well. . . This can show up as a weak or ambiguous orgasm, an uncomfortable orgasm, or no orgasm altogether." Fritchle also says that SSRIs may cause loss of sensation and sometimes numbness in the nipples and genitals.

Trusted primary care physician Sarah Fang, DO, strongly believes that when it comes to SSRIs, it's important for doctors to explain the potential side effects because many of them can lead to sexual, physiological, or emotional shifts, and it's imperative to know SSRIs aren't the only medications that affect sexuality. Beta-blockers, used to treat high blood pressure and certain heart problems, as well as plenty of other nonpsychotropic medications, can also affect sexual functioning. If you're trans and undergoing gender-affirming hormone therapy, those treatments will likely affect your sexual experience as well.

If you're taking a medication with sexual side effects, and your sexuality matters to you, you will need to have open, honest discussions with your trusted medical professionals about your needs, sexual and otherwise. If your doctor isn't openly asking you about sex or if talking about sex is challenging for you, you are not alone, and these conversations can be extremely tough to have. However, as Fritchle affirms, "you have to be the one to advocate for yourself and say, 'Not only am I experiencing this, but sexuality is important to me,' because a lot of doctors may treat sex with indifference," especially if you don't tell them it's something you value. It's important to initiate difficult conversations about medications and sexuality to ensure that your mental *and* sexual needs are met. If you find yourself in this position and have not done so already, it's highly advised you have dialogue with your trusted medical professional before making any (further) decisions about your medication(s).

Dr. Fang emphasizes that this open sharing only helps all parties involved: "Our role as physicians is to help you make decisions to be the healthiest version of yourself. Part of that may be where your mental health and sexual health intersect. We are not there to judge your character or sexual concerns. Be transparent with your doctor so they can partner with you to meet your health goals."

 Gain more confidence in talking to your medical professional about medication and sex in episode #113, "Depression, Anxiety, SSRIs, and Sex—with Melissa Fritchle, LMFT."

When Pleasure Becomes Challenging

If you've experienced a shift in your mind or body's response to sexuality, be sure to consider all the factors contributing to your well-being. This includes your relationships (or lack thereof) with your partner(s), as well as with your family, friends, kids, colleagues, and anyone who has an impact on you. However, it also includes your work life, financial stability, mental and physical health, feelings about the world, and the current state of the environment. All of these things can impact your sexuality.

Through her extensive work on "delayed ejaculation," the term for situations where orgasm is seemingly difficult or even unobtainable, Keeley Rankin, MA, has developed a set of tools for rediscovering pleasure when pleasure has become a challenge (she even offers full-scale online courses on it). Though Rankin is known for her focus on supporting penis owners, these tools apply to vulva owners too.

Keeley Rankin's Tools for Rediscovering Pleasure

1. **Take the habit out of pleasure**. Start with changing up the way you're masturbating and expanding the ways in which you can find orgasm. Sometimes there's a particular way you're touching your body that conditions your brain. Maybe it's watching porn or playing with toys—it's where pleasure becomes a habit. In regard to fantasies, if you always go to a specific place in your head to find your orgasm, relearning how to achieve pleasure is about figuring out what your actual turn-ons are and how you move into those with your own body (or a partner) without always going into that

familiar fantasy. Learn how to diversify your body's ability to take in and receive pleasure and ask yourself what your needs and wants really are.

2. **Take a pleasure inventory**. Is porn a part of your regular pleasure practice? Consider taking a break from porn for a few weeks while continuing a self-pleasure practice to see if this plays a role in your sexual shift. Are sex toys your go-to pleasure object of choice? Perhaps see what sex and masturbation would be like without those things for a while. Additionally, take an inventory of what's happened in your life around the time of the shift. Did something change in your emotional world that affected your ability to let go and feel safe? This may include anything from a life-changing experience, like heartbreak or grief, to smaller yet still impactful experiences such as, for example, a failure to orgasm that led you down a rabbit hole of self-doubt and criticism—maybe compounded by a critical comment from your partner that only intensified that internalized pressure. And the last thing to check for in your inventory: Do you feel safety and trust around sex, with your partner(s) or yourself? This is key.

3. **Build trust and safety**. Trust plays an immense role in the ability to let go during sex. Ask yourself: *What does it mean to lose control?* Because essentially, releasing into orgasm is a loss of control. Your body reacts, makes noises, perhaps you make faces; there are all sorts of things that can happen, and it has a lot to do with the question of: *How much do you trust?* Can you let yourself release into this space and just be okay with what's going to happen? Trust is necessary whether or not you've ever orgasmed, and whether or not you're

with a partner—each situation requires its own kind of trust in the unknown. If your inventory tells you safety and trust are a part of the issue, then maybe it's time to make some strong commitments to yourself and/or have conversations with your partner(s) so they're aware of your process. What if orgasming during sex was taken off the table for a while, and the only goal was pleasure? What if orgasm was just a bonus, and all the other fun, sensual experiences that happen along the way became the primary focus? Concentrate on your needs and what brings you closest to meeting them, rather than pre-set expectations.

 Rethink your ideas about orgasm and pleasure by listening to episode #199, "All About ORGASMS—with Keeley Rankin."

In addition to these helpful tools, we'd also encourage you to explore finding new ways to play. This can be especially helpful if your body is changing so much that the old ways you used to experience pleasure or orgasm feel unobtainable. But even if that's not the case for you—it is always fun to try new things! We'll be suggesting some tips for creating newness as we answer the next sex question but, because novelty is such a foundational part of sex and relationships, we dedicated all of Chapter 7 to that very topic.

I WANT TO CONTINUE EXPERIENCING SEXUAL PLEASURE BUT MY BODY DOESN'T SEEM TO ALLOW IT

I had a life-saving surgery, and as a result my sex drive dropped to the point of non-existence. I push myself to have sex every few weeks, but the entire time I am thinking about how I would rather be sleeping. As you can imagine, my partner feels rejected, and I feel bad for putting my partner through this. I am working with a wonderful doctor trying to get my hormones balanced, but so far we aren't there yet. I want to satisfy my partner's needs, but I feel like I don't know how to anymore. We have listened to your podcast and know masturbation is an option, but it still leaves my partner feeling unfulfilled. Is there anything I can do to change or am I just damaged goods?

People of all genders and orientations are conditioned to caretake their partner's sexual wants and desires. This is often a symptom of upbringing, perhaps from seeing one parent doing the majority of the caretaking in the family. It could also go back to childhood socialization, when helping others before yourself might have also helped you achieve acceptance or maintain a sense of belonging. Or maybe it could have come from mainstream media, which generally equates true love with choosing your partner's needs over your own. But don't worry, there are ways to address this caretaking behavior to ensure that everyone involved gets a fair shot at experiencing pleasure.

The Orgasm Gap

Though it's not exclusive to this context by any means, the concern being addressed in this sex question—namely, the need to satisfy a partner's needs before your own—seems to occur most frequently with cis women in relationships with cis men. In Western culture, this is probably due to centuries of erroneous myths and teachings about vulva owners', specifically women's, sexuality, combined with gender prejudices about subordinating their pleasure to men's, putting cis women involved with cis men in the crosshairs of these stereotypes—though they also certainly remain in play for people of other gender experiences.

Some of the most frequent offenders are about sex drive. Stereotypes would have you believe that vulva owners naturally have a lower sex drive than penis owners. This is complete bullshit! In her incredible book *Untrue: Why Nearly Everything We Believe About Women, Lust, and Infidelity Is Wrong and How the New Science Can Set Us Free*, sexuality expert Wednesday Martin, PhD, explains, "The female libido, when measured correctly, is every bit as strong as the male. Women are sexually weirder than we ever thought—and that's normal!"

 Free yourself from the orgasm gap with episode #82, "The Truth About Women, Lust, and Adultery—with Wednesday Martin, PhD."

Cultural prejudices (often in heterosexual relationships) also dictate that if a vulva owner has a *lower* sex drive than their penis-owning partner, they are the ones who should change to feel more aroused. Conversely, if the vulva owner has a *higher* sex drive than their penis-owning partner, they are often deemed as "slutty" or the one with the problem. These notions are biased and need to be dismantled. In her book *Come As You Are*, Emily Nagoski, PhD, highlights these myths' origins in a penis-centric model of sexuality, which has been forcing cis women in particular to view themselves through a scope that not only wasn't made for them but which also perpetuates false ideas. All of these beliefs deserve the middle finger and a wave goodbye.

Hormones and Sexuality

We've said it before, and we'll say it again: People change all the time, because of age, health, environment, and many other reasons, and this is completely normal. However, modern medicine allows us to have more and more choice in these changes. Urology specialist Dr. Lamia Gabal gives a few examples of this: "It's normal for breasts to change as people get older, and we have breast augmentation and breast lifts we can do if that's important to you. It's also normal for people's testosterone to go down as they get older, and we have something called bioidentical hormone pelleting that we offer in our practice as well." For those dealing with menopause, Dr. Gabal identifies, "bioidentical hormone replacements . . . put into the fat by a little injection once every few months" as an option that "mimics more of what your body used to make when you were younger or before your hormones changed."

Hormones are responsible for a *lot* of your life as a sexual being. Estrogen, for example, "is in charge of so many things . . . including libido, a sense of well-being, even the quality of the hair, skin, [genitals], and so on," says Dr. Gabal. Additionally, "For all genders we have 'normal' amounts of testosterone, [which] change with age," and which (among other hormones) affect sensation in vulvas, penises, and all the in-betweens. But fortunately, "we now have the option to optimize hormones . . . [which can result] in enhanced sexual enjoyment and sexual function."

Non-hormonal options for optimizing sexual health are also growing. Procedures such as the O-shot (injecting the clitoris and labia with platelet-rich plasma) and the P-shot (a similar injection but for the penis), as well as FemiWave and GAINSWave (which use pulse waves to improve blood flow to sexual organs), all serve to enhance sensation and blood flow in the genitals, according to urologist and *Shameless Sex* guest Dr. Nicole Eisenbrown.

 Learn about the current medical advances in sexual optimization in episodes #169, "Sex, Aging, and Urology—with Dr. Lamia Gabal," and #240, "How to Stop Having Painful Sex & Sexual Dysfunction—with urologist Dr. Nicole Eisenbrown."

Keep in mind that scientific knowledge of sexual health and wellness is constantly advancing. By the time you finish reading this book, experts may have already discovered completely different understandings about the ideas we shared here. There may also be a plethora of exciting innovations and new technologies available that we haven't even mentioned here—that's why we encourage you to use this information as a starting point for your own research. We'll be your personal cheerleaders every step of the way, pom-poms and all.

Get Multiple Opinions Before Making Big Decisions

If it's within your financial means, consider seeing multiple doctors to get a few different perspectives and opinions about your body's sexual function. As is the case with therapists, friends, partners, and lovers, not all doctors will be the right fit for you. Your relationship with your doctor is professional yet intimate, and it's important to work with someone who makes you feel safe, understood, and capable of pursuing your unique goals. And remember: *You are not broken or damaged.* You are unique and beautiful, and pleasure is your birthright.

I WANT TO CONTINUE EXPERIENCING SEXUAL PLEASURE BUT MY BODY DOESN'T SEEM TO ALLOW IT

1. Do you want to learn how to talk to your partner about the shifts in your body and what might work better for you to enjoy sex? If so, continue to read this chapter. We also recommend going to page **148** of **Chapter 4: How Can I Ask for What I Want or Even Talk About Sex?** for navigating challenging conversations around sex.

2. Would you like to expand your definition of sex to include options beyond the sex you're currently having? If so, continue to read this chapter. We also recommend reading page **234** of **Chapter 7: How Can I Have a Hotter, Steamier, More Connected Sex Life?** for alternative ways to turn up the heat in the bedroom.

3. Do you want to get clear on what you need as a sexual being? If so, read **Chapter 3: How Do I Know What I Want in the Bedroom?** for gaining a better understanding around knowing what you desire in sex.

The Power of AND

Change is a part of being human that can be a blessing and a curse. If you are the type of person who meets change with resistance, approaching with the mindset of *I do not want this. I do not like this. I will not accept this*—you're not alone, and we completely get you. But this perspective often only brings *more* inner turmoil to your physical and emotional states.

Even though it's hard, there is another option to choose and this includes the word "and." Here is an example: *I do not want this, I do not like this, AND here's where I am now, AND how can I explore my options to work with what is true in this moment AND embrace what is and what isn't.* Inviting "and" into your perspective opens up opportunities to reassess where you once were and your attachment to that place, while also taking in the now and considering how to move forward in a way that feels helpful, manageable, and even deeply fulfilling for you. Many *Shameless Sex* listeners who have taken this difficult step have shared that accepting the present and opening themselves to new possibilities has actually resulted in stronger connections and more profound sex. It may not be what they thought it would (or should) be, yet they are having some of the best intimate experiences of their lives.

Finding New Ways to Play

One of the most common prescriptions for these types of transformations does not involve medication or surgery. Instead, they are available to almost everyone with openness to this crucial tool. Find new ways to play! Whether this means combining your usual sexual activities with something new, or crossing off old activities from your sexual menu entirely and adding separate new actions and behaviors, finding new ways to play makes the possibilities for reinventing your personal sexual wheel limitless. This novelty can be incredibly helpful in adapting to lots of different situations, from medical, health and ability, and hormonal changes, to the inevitable processes of aging. This can even be helpful for those experiencing gender dysphoria around sex or their bits.

For those in a situation like the one described in this sex question, what if your body simply needs more or less of something then it did before your body changed (in this case, due to the medical procedure)? Perhaps penetration is still on the menu, but your system now needs ten times more slowness, love, care, and even nonsexual touch. Consider the possibility that penetration may be a no-go for you at this point—but maybe your external bits are a yes to hands, mouths, and even sex toys. This is an invitation for you—and everyone—to expand your definition of what sex means to you, particularly regarding what feels good for you now.

Shameless Sex Tips to Reinvent Your Definition of Sex

- **Redefine sex** as something outside of penetration or any other pre-set notions of what sex should be. Can a long make-out session be a part of sex, even when it doesn't lead to anything more? What about a sensual massage involving rubbing parts of your body besides your genitals? Or can an erotic massage include well-lubed hands slowly kneading the external genitals—without penetration at all? Can sex include pleasurable activities with a soft penis, or arousing play that doesn't involve or expect orgasm?

- **Erotic massage** is a great practice for folks with receiving barriers—where an internal struggle results in feelings like *I'm taking too long, I need to do something to pleasure my partner,* or *It's not okay for this to just be about me,* etc. Receiving barriers are quite common, especially for folks who feel like their partner's pleasure takes priority over their own. Hence why it's a "massage" and not a "handjob"—the former implies relaxation, pleasure, even healing, while the other points to an agenda where pleasure is expected to result in orgasm.

- **Foreplay** is your best friend. If you're with a partner (or partners), just because one person is aroused does not mean the other(s) are! This can be especially relevant in the case of sex between vulva owners and penis owners: according to Nagoski, engorgement and arousal take approximately four times as long for most vulvas as for most penises. If your body has changed recently, you may need more foreplay than you did previously. This can involve sensual touch or non-touch-based sources of arousal, such as watching porn, reading or listening to erotica (check out our favorite app for that, Dipsea), or connecting with your partner in a way that speaks to your unique sexual language.

- With any **oral sex** and **hand sex** (handjobs), remind yourself that it doesn't need to lead to anything more and it can be its own sexy isolated event. With hand sex in particular, make sure you feel warmed up and aroused—especially if it involves internal stimulation. Since your genitals are mucous membranes, they generally prefer to be touched with well-lubricated fingers and hands, so be sure to have some good lube nearby too (we love überlube!).

- Try **dry humping** (grinding bodies against each other) with or without clothing—which can even end up being more arousing than genital-on-genital sex itself.

- Try exploring **non-ejaculatory sex** (if you or your partner is a penis owner). This generally involves learning how to orgasm in new ways without expelling your fluids, and while a lot people find it hard to master, it can also be a life-changing addition to your sexual menu— as age-old traditions like Taoism and Tantra recognize.

 Discover the how-tos of non-ejaculatory sex with episode #260, "Semen Retention and Becoming the Master of Your Cock—with Fabienne Annike."

- Use **sex toys**. Sex toys can be a game changer not only for solo play but also for partnered play. You can use toys on your own body in front of your partner, building up arousal before connecting with another body, or you can use them to simultaneously stimulate your bits in front of each other. Once you have your sex toy game down, you can also incorporate them into other sexual activities with your partner (Chapter 3 will help you master your sex toy game).

As an extra piece of encouragement: redefining your definition of sex while re-creating your yeses, nos, and maybes for this newfound sexual menu can be fun, exciting, and sexy. It depends on how you approach it, as well as your partner's willingness to work with you. You may also uncover that this process will invite your partner to share more about their own yeses, nos, and maybes. When you fully share yourself and lovingly lead by example, you are also giving your partner the permission to do the same for themself. And that's something that should give you a big smile.

What Does Sexy Mean to YOU?

Everyone's experience of sexuality is unique, and sex drive is no different. Sex drive can, however, be affected by what bits and hormones you've got going on. Because higher testosterone levels are connected to a higher *spontaneous* sex drive, or a feeling of "craving" sex, people with more testosterone—including, often but not exclusively, many penis owners—are more likely to experience this type of drive toward sex. Meanwhile, the hormone cocktails commonly occurring in the bodies of many vulva owners can make them more likely to experience a *responsive* sex drive, which means that these bodies need more sensation and connection to get into their turn-on, or they require some action to arouse their bits (though, of course, this experience is by no means exclusive to vulva owners). Arousal patterns often change within people and even within relationships over time.

For Amy, just hearing how important she is to her partner during a moment of deep loving connection can get her pussy pulsating all on its own. In fact, her sex drive is almost always responsive as opposed to spontaneous, regardless of how long she's been in the relationship. April, on the other hand, often gets turned on just by seeing naked bodies or thinking about sex and dirty talk. She has a more spontaneous sex drive, even in long-term relationships.

Sexologist Jaiya's Erotic Blueprints provide an innovative way to discover more about your own turn-ons and the ins and outs of your desire patterns in episode #126, "Erotic Blueprints—with Jaiya."

YOUR JOURNEY IS YOURS

Remember, no matter who you are or what you've experienced on your journey of life, *you are not broken!* Yes, there may be times when you feel that way, but just know that there is nothing wrong with you as a sexual being. It's understandable that sometimes you may want to deny or dismiss things by telling yourself to "just get over it" and move on—that's a common response to traumatic experiences. Don't let the urge to dismiss things prevent you from pursuing what you need and want in your sexuality. You are worthy of the pursuit.

We hope that this chapter—and this whole book—can help you explore your feelings and find more ways to feel more connected to yourself, your relationships, and the world around you. Your journey is yours, and so are the struggles you've faced, no matter how big or small. But they don't have to define you or dictate who you are as a sexual being. You have the power and the pencil to write your own sexy story—with whatever beginning, middle, and end you desire.

How Do I Know What I Want in the Bedroom?

We know—identifying what you want sexually is hard. It requires developing your understanding of your individual needs and even exploring why there could be blocks keeping you from accessing your ultimate desires (or even your full knowledge of them). Of course, you'll also need to develop the skills to ask for what you want, which we'll cover in Chapter 4. But first, you need to become an archaeologist of the self so you can excavate and examine the intricacies of your own sexual being. Consider this chapter the lube that preps you for entering the next chapter. You could skip it, but that would probably create a lot of uncomfortable friction.

WHY IS IT SO HARD TO KNOW WHAT YOU WANT?

Even if you're a person who knows a great deal about your inner erotic landscape or are satisfied with what's happening in the bedroom right now, your sexual and relationship needs are still apt to change as time passes, just like your body and perspective. As a result, it's common for anyone to occasionally feel stuck or disconnected from their sexuality. Fear not, because this chapter is here to help you break free from that rut time and time again.

As we've discussed, your brain and your cultural and societal conditioning play a pivotal role in how you think about sex. The world's suggestions about what you should want or need (especially in order to be "normal") in the bedroom are powerful, and the shame and trauma that they can cause may lead your mind, body, and spirit to put up protective walls during intimate experiences with yourself and others. Another effect of living with constant pressure to conform to norms is people-pleasing: a (sub)conscious survival tactic that seems helpful at first glance, yet only complicates the confusing labyrinth of discovering your true sexual essence.

THE DECEPTIVE ART OF PEOPLE-PLEASING

Amy, a self-proclaimed people pleaser, has repeatedly prioritized the sexual needs of her partners at the expense of her own needs. This behavior can be attributed, in part, to inadequate sex ed and awareness of the importance of her own sexual pleasure (thank you, US public school system) and the necessity of exploring and understanding her body and what it desired before sharing it with others.

Another important factor was her gender conditioning. As Peggy Orenstein shares in her book *Girls & Sex: Navigating the Complicated New Landscape*, people socialized as women (especially with the expectation of future heterosexual partnerships) are often conditioned to take on a caretaker role in relationships. Kate Loree, LMFT, affirms this, noting that most women or girls have been groomed by society to overgive, take care of others, and forfeit needs as a means of supporting their romantic partners. Instead of discovering what feels good to them, they put their partners' pleasure above their own, while simultaneously waiting for their partners to show them what they should enjoy sexually. This type of habituation has been going on for hundreds and hundreds of years and is very detrimental to the process of uncovering one's unique sexual desires.

 Empower yourself with more tools to start choosing *you* in episode #301, "Narcissism and Healing After Toxic Relationships—With Kate Loree, LMFT"

April is also no stranger to deprioritizing her sexual needs either. From her teens to her late twenties, April only knew what orgasm felt like from masturbation sessions that were shadowed by shame. That, combined with lots of awkward, orgasmless sexual experiences, caused her to train herself to fake orgasms so her partners would cum faster and believe they were amazing in the bedroom. She never talked about her sexual needs, likes, or dislikes because she didn't want to risk losing a lover's interest or affection (nor did she think her pleasure mattered). Clearly, this was unsustainable. When April couldn't repress her erotic desires any longer, she finally started the process of uncovering them for herself (not for anyone else). Once she finally tapped into her desire and began honoring herself in sexual exchanges, the number on her sexual

Richter scale was off the charts. She didn't need to fake her orgasms anymore because she wasn't trying to get the sex part over with—it was just that damn pleasurable.

But don't get it twisted, people-pleasing isn't exclusive to those socialized as women. Anyone can be vulnerable to getting sucked into the vortex of compliant sex that doesn't reflect their wants or needs. But the beauty of it all is that with time, dedication, and some conscious effort, everyone—including *you*—can discover who they are as a sexual being and get all that yummy yummy good stuff they want in the bedroom.

I DON'T KNOW WHAT I WANT DURING SEX

I was raised in a family where sex was never talked about. I'm in a relationship with someone who likes sex and is more open about it than me. I'm scared I won't be able to keep my partner interested. When I hear "What do you want and what are your fantasies?" I just draw a blank because I really have no idea and usually respond with "What do you want?"—resulting in frustration from my partner. I want to try different things and be more assertive, but I don't know how to do that. I like penetrative sex, but I don't orgasm during it, and I end up in my head because I know my partner wants me to. How can I learn more about my body, what I want, and get confident about sharing these kinds of things?

If you struggle with knowing what you want during sex, the reasons can be multilayered. But a big one for anyone raised in a traditional or conservative religious environment is that they may have negative and shameful views concerning sex. So it's not surprising that a lot people reach adulthood without a clue about their own bodies and what brings them pleasure, especially when they lack the necessary resources and knowledge to advocate for themselves. Some are fortunate enough to have received "comprehensive sex education" where they learn about anatomy, safer-sex practices, consent, and other clinical aspects of sexuality. But when it comes to pleasure and how to explore the body by finding techniques for self-pleasuring and sharing touch with others, it is completely understandable to not know what's going on, or to stumble through learning on your own through trial and error. If this sounds like you, we are with you, and we want to help!

Your Bits Are Unique and There Is No One-Size-Fits-All Approach

We firmly believe that sex must take place in a setting that values mutual pleasure and respect for each other's boundaries and differences. This requires a shift in mindset from prioritizing others' needs over your own, despite what societal norms may have taught you.

Furthermore, each person in a sexual encounter is always going to have a completely unique set of needs—even on the physical level alone. For example, in the previous chapter, we mentioned that vulvas, on average, take about four times longer to become aroused than penises. As another receiving orifice, the anus is similar—it requires extra time and warm-up, and pleasurable anal sex depends on the receiver's ability to relax and open up. This is quite the opposite of what the penetrating partner needs to do! So remember that your needs are unique to you, as are your bits—which themselves are distinct from all the other billions of people's bits on this planet (and on other planets too).

Unless your partner is psychic, they will not automatically have the perfect blueprint to attend to your body's specific sexual needs. They can listen to every podcast and read all the books on sexual mastery in the world and still never know what your body desires. Therefore, it is imperative to take the time to explore your own body. If you have no idea where to start—don't worry! We'll make sure you have the basics down by the end of this chapter.

Porn and Sexuality

Before we move on to the amazing things you can learn by exploring your body (and how to do it), let's briefly discuss *bad* sex ed . . . namely, porn. Hopefully, we aren't the first people to tell you that most pornography is designed for entertainment, not education. It can be a great tool for gaining inspiration about your turn-ons, but not for learning "how to do sex." In fact, most porn is pretty inaccurate to real life—especially in how it depicts the receiver of penetration, who often needs more connection and warm-up than is shown. This depiction makes sense, though—since porn is designed to turn the viewer on and profit off their arousal (and corresponding dopamine production from their brain), it's a smart business move to try to get that dopamine flowing as intensely and as quickly as possible.

If you're surprised by this information because you've only been in the role of the penetrator, we have some homework for you: Do some R&D on yourself so you can better understand the people you're playing with. Try inserting the tip of a *well-lubed* finger into the universal orifice—your asshole—and see how long it takes before your ass is ready to let you in further. (Hint: it can take a while.)

If viewing porn is new to you, remind yourself that the people get-ting sexy on screen are well-trained actors and sexual athletes (shout out to porn performers—we respect, appreciate, and honor you!), and the way you have sex does *not* need to replicate what they're doing.

 Discover the importance of the receiver coming first by listening to episodes #167, "She Comes First—with Ian Kerner, PhD," and #44, "Sexual Mastery: Pussies, Vulvas, Yonis—with Amy and April"

And now, it's time to dust off your archaeology pants and gloves (get that khaki-colored hat out too while you're at it!) so you can dig deep and sift through these Pleasure Paths to uncover what you want in the bedroom.

I DON'T KNOW WHAT I WANT DURING SEX

1. Do you want to develop a better understanding of what your body likes and dislikes so you can discover things that you want to try in the bedroom? If so, continue to read this chapter. We also rec-ommend going to page **206** of **Chapter 6: How Can I Become a Better Lover?** or page **36** of **Chapter 1: Am I Normal?** to learn why many vulva owners are not having orgasms during penetrative sex and uncover key tools to help shift that. Also, reading pages **58** and **65** of **Chapter 2: Am I Broken?** which discuss seek-ing pleasure after shame, trauma, or other difficult situations, might be helpful.

2. Do you think shame and/or trauma could be affecting your connection with your partner? Or do you have an internal belief that this is your fault or there is something wrong with you? If so, we recommend going back to page **29** in **Chapter 1: Am I Normal?** to understand how to work with shame and trauma and learn ways to shift limiting beliefs. Also, go back to page **58** in **Chapter 2: Am I Broken?** to discern why those blocks exist and how to move through them.

3. Would you like some direction on how to clearly convey your desires to your partner? If so, reading the CONNECT formula on page **148** of **Chapter 4: How Can I Ask for What I Want or Even Talk About Sex?** will help with communication when having difficult conversations around sex.

4. Are you interested in learning about new ways to play and various types of "adventurous" sex or fantasies you could explore? If so, check out page **234** in **Chapter 7: How Can I Have a Hotter, Steamier, More Connected Sex Life?**, which provides a multitude of options for sexual exploration in these departments.

Self-Pleasure Is Your New Bestie

If you're looking to absorb more information about your sexual being, then consider self-pleasure the ultimate sponge. One of the first things to consider is your self-pleasure practice and masturbation history. Have you ever taken the time to explore your body through solo sex? That's masturbation, rubbing one out, batin', shining the clam, wanking, or flogging the dolphin in the safety of your own space without anyone present. If your answer is no, then get ready for plenty of tips on how to begin your self-pleasure journey—because it's one of the best things you can do for your sexual well-being, and it's your ticket for having great sex with your partner(s).

Maybe your answer is yes, but you still sense that you haven't unlocked the full extent of your body's pleasure potential. Don't hold back now, because we have a trove of tips and tricks so you can excavate your erotic terrain and unleash the pleasure hidden within in that gorgeous body of yours. Whether you lack experience, have confusion around the body's inner workings, or even have performance anxiety, you're not alone— these are all common barriers for a lot of people. For example, one memorable day while Amy and April were working in Pure Pleasure Shop's retail store, they met an eighty-year-old woman who came in to purchase her very first vibrator after her husband of sixty years passed away. Although she'd been partnered for a very long time, she had never experienced an orgasm. She didn't know if she liked internal or external pleasure, and she wasn't sure if she could even have an orgasm, but she left that day with her very first vibrator. Three weeks later, she returned with tears in her eyes to deliver a thank you card that expressed her gratitude for "changing her life forever" because she had finally experienced her first orgasm from the curved G-spot toy she had purchased. This beautiful story exemplifies why exploring your body on your own by taking pleasure into your own hands—at any age—is so incredibly important.

Practice Self-Pleasure Like It's a Dance

Some masturbation newbies will discover the intricate ways they prefer to be touched or what leads them to orgasm within a few sessions. And some won't. For those who have been sexually active for many years, the process will probably take more time and dedication. This is why it's called a self-pleasure *practice*—it's not a one-and-done kind of thing. It involves making a commitment to caring for yourself, discovering your body, and allocating time to practice what you've learned. It's like learning how to salsa dance. The first time feels challenging and even dissatisfying. But what if you went to that salsa class every day for a week or five times a week for a month? You would get comfortable with the movements, better understand the techniques, and feel more confident with every class you attended.

When it comes to your sexuality, you're still "going to class," but in the comfort and privacy of your own space, with just your mind, body, and maybe some sex toys. You're the person in charge, utilizing the expertise you've gathered beforehand. If it feels like a chore, remind yourself that this "work" will ultimately lead to easier and more pleasurable sex—it's an investment in you. Plus, taking care of your sexuality is like giving yourself a present that benefits your entire well-being. It really is the gift that keeps on giving.

Here are some tips to get you geared up to scale that mountain of pleasure existing within your body.

Shameless Sex's Ways to Stimulate Self-Pleasure

1. **Take time.** Designate solo time to discover what pleases your body. If you'd like some guidance on what to do after you've set aside that time, go back to page **41** of **Chapter 1: Am I Normal?** and check out "*Shameless Sex*'s Tips for Uncovering Your O" because it has some great advice on ways to get sexy with thyself.

2. **Get into the zone.** Your self-pleasure zone needs to feel safe and free of any interruptions. If you get stuck in your head easily, set a timer so you can sit back, relax, and not worry about keeping track of when the session will end.

3. **Set the scene.** Create an environment that inspires relaxation and sensuality. Think about what music to play, the type of sexy lighting you want (like candles or a red light bulb in a lamp), the clothes you're wearing or not wearing, the areas where the session will take place (for instance, on the bed, in front of the mirror, or in the bathtub). Design a scene that will support you as you drop into your sexual essence.

4. **Traverse with touch.** Begin to explore your body by going *slower than slow, and then slower than that.* Mindfully observe all the subtleties of sensation that you experience. Identify the areas where you feel hints of pleasure, warmth, or tingling, and stay with those sensations for awhile before diving deeper. If you encounter discomfort, numbness, or any other unpleasant sensations, try to get curious about those parts of your body—but only if it feels safe. Notice where you feel these sensations and the type of touch, level of pressure, and the speed at which they activate. Experiment with different types of touch such as less pressure, slower tempo, or even a brief pause to see what feels best. Listen to the messages your body is trying to convey to understand your likes and dislikes. Once you become familiar with what touch your body wants, share your discoveries with your partner (if you have one) before your next sexy-time session to guide them to touch you in the ways that you prefer.

5. **Explore just about everywhere.** Invite your hands to move all over your body as slowly as possible and pay attention to any sensation that

arises. Maybe your hands are placed over your belly or gently rubbing your inner thighs. Perhaps you're touching your nipples and testing out various forms of pressure and speed. Or maybe your hands are on your genitals, rubbing, massaging, and tapping different parts. The possibilities are endless—just allow your hands to be the intuitive conductors of your body's desires and you could discover things you never knew about your body. If you need more examples of possible ways to explore the vulva, check out OMGyes.com.

6. **Get inspired by porn.** Porn can serve as a mechanism to introduce you to new themes, categories, or actions that get your bits throbbing. There is infinite content available on the internet, but pause for a moment of consideration before you begin entering keywords into the search engine. Think about what you want or don't want. You could watch something that doesn't sit right with you, resulting in a complex shame spiral. If this happens, add whatever you viewed to your "I don't like" list on your sexual menu and follow up with self-care (for ideas, revisit Chapter 2). As a reminder, while porn can offer inspiration, it's designed for entertainment and not education.

It's also important to keep in mind that adult performers are real human beings, and porn is the way they financially provide for themselves. The free content online generally does not adequately compensate the time and energy that performers put into what you're viewing. If you find yourself watching someone on a free site and you want to continue watching that particular performer, consider paying to get your wank on via their preferred platforms, so their skills can earn them the money they deserve.

7. **Journal your journey.** After each self-pleasure session, write down what you've discovered by noting the areas and ways your body liked or disliked your touch. Also, write down how you were feeling before you entered the session. What was your stress level? How did you sleep the previous night? Did you exercise that day? Were there any outside factors impacting your emotional state? Then, note how you feel after the session. Are there any noticeable shifts or changes in your mood? Get curious about the before and after.

8. **Circle back and revisit.** Each time you practice, look back at the pleasure notes you took from the previous session and see if there's a place to focus on during this round. Do your notes suggest a particularly effective method of touch on a certain area of your bits? Was there an uncomfortable zone that you'd like to avoid? Maybe your notes suggest more rapidity and pressure when you're having a hard day. Your masturbation practice can be informative, dynamic, and always evolving. Savor all of these nuances and let your growing knowledge and understanding guide you as you move forward into other sexual experiences, solo or otherwise.

9. **Experiment with sex toys.** Welcome to the wonderful world of wanking with sex toys! We're giddy with every exclamation of excitement possible—yippee, hurray, woo-hoo, yee-haw, and fuck yeah! There are reasons to believe humans have used objects other than bodies to get off since the dawn of humanity. But we can say with full confidence that the golden age of sex toys is *now*—with countless advances in sex tech and massive improvements in product innovation, accessing the right toys has never been easier. It only takes a quick peek at what the first vibrators looked like to appreciate

how much progress has been made in the century since they were invented. We can't wait to spread our good vibes your way because sex toys are a *Shameless Sex* obsession, and we'll come back to them in a sexy second.

If you found yourself particularly turned-on or curious about anything you've learned from practicing these tips, add those to your list of things "I might want to try" on your sexual menu. This doesn't mean you have to act anything out in real time—it could be something that works to arouse you only by thinking or talking about it. If you're with a partner, sometimes simply sharing those naughty turn-ons with them is all you need to add a little spice into your sexual soup.

Choosing the Right Sex Toy (for Vulva Owners)

Before you can enjoy the marvels of sex toys, you have to answer an important question: What's the right sex toy for you? It's amazing that there are so many possibilities available, but this can lead to severe option anxiety and overwhelm when it comes to shopping for yourself—not to mention if you want something for you and your partner(s). For this reason, we recommend bringing your questions to sex-positive adult shops and pleasure boutiques, where the staff are well-trained in understanding the products and well prepared to help you find which product is best suited for your needs.

If you do not have access to a nearby sex-positive retail store (or if you're just nervous—though we're pretty certain sex shop employees don't bite), shop online instead. Many sex-positive e-commerce retailers (like purepleasureshop.com) allow you to ask questions and share what you're looking for via email where trained staff members will respond with product recommendations. Some sites even offer live chat messaging, so you can discuss your questions in real time.

If you're a vulva owner, getting yourself a vibrator is a great place to start expanding your pleasure potential. Because the clitoris (for reference, see the diagram on page 38) is the primary pleasure zone for vulva owners, it's likely that the external genitals will be a self-pleasure area of focus for you.

This is why you may want to consider starting with a vibrator designed for external use and not for insertion. Many of these vibes come in smaller sizes, which makes them easier to incorporate into sexy time with your partner(s), if you decide to do that. Amy loves products with air-pulse technology which provide a type of suction sensation that feels powerful yet not overwhelming. Meanwhile, April is more of a "power queen"—she loves high-powered products that deliver deep frequency vibrations. For her, nothing beats a wand-style massager like the Magic Wand. Another go-to is a compact multi-speed vibrator, like Hot Octopuss's AMO and DiGiT—small enough to travel with but still able to provide the powerful vibrations she needs from a sex toy.

However, some people love the sensation of internal penetration alongside the external vibrations. If this sounds titillating to you, then choose an internal vibe, or a "rabbit" style designed for dual (internal and external) stimulation. For internal/G-area exploration, April prefers the KURVE by Hot Octopuss because of its squishy tip and two independent motors (one is deep and rumbly while the other is high pitched and buzzy, so you can navigate to find exactly the right frequency for your bits). Amy

Examples of External Vibrators

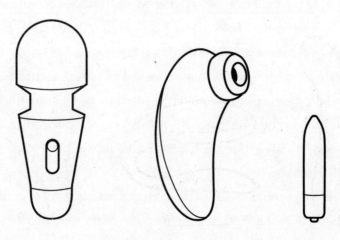

doesn't really prefer internal vibrations, but her mom Janis's favorites are the Miss Bi and Amorino by Fun Factory because they offer some of the best quality motors on the market that simultaneously deliver internal and clitoral stimulation.

Whichever type of vibe you choose, make sure the toy is made from body-safe materials like silicone or ABS plastic, which are both nonporous (to inhibit bacterial growth) and easy to clean. We'd also recommend a vibe that has multiple speed options. When you begin playing with your toy, start with the lowest level of vibration intensity to avoid overwhelming your genitals with this brand-new sensation.

Think of finding your ideal sex toy like you're exploring a pleasure-filled theme park. Each attraction you decide to ride on will be very different. Some rides you'll enjoy a handful of times but then you may get bored, while others can feel strange or uncomfortable. And then there's

Examples of Internal Vibrators

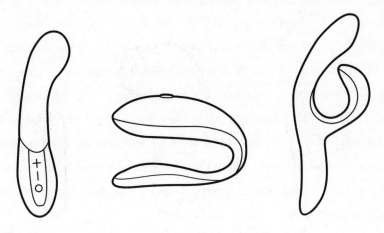

the fabulous few that will absolutely blow your mind again and again. The only thing is, you have to take the ride to know which is your favorite—so now it's about time to buy the ticket and hop on the ride!

Myth-Busting Vibes

You may be hesitant to use a vibrator—and that's fine. Always do what feels best for you. But we must clear up two common misconceptions about using vibrators just in case your hesitation is based on either of them. Misconception #1 is the idea that you can somehow become "addicted" to a vibrator. Well, you can't. Vibrators work just like any other pleasurable activity: by releasing oxytocin and dopamine in your brain. It's true that continual use can cause your brain and body to link the vibrator to that pleasurable release—but only in the same way that the brain can habituate to *any* repeated stimuli. So don't worry, you won't have to go through any vibe "withdrawals" anytime soon. These toys are just an easy way to get yourself to O Town.

Now let's confront misconception #2: that vibrators will desensitize your bits. This is a total myth. It is possible some people will experience a temporary numbing sensation after using high-powered vibrators, but this goes away within hours. A study from *The Journal of Sexual Medicine* found that most vibrators have no adverse effects whatsoever on the genitals—and in fact there's actually a tremendous amount of evidence correlating the use of vibrators with positive sexual health benefits such as increased blood flow and arousal.

In truth, if you're able to orgasm from using a vibrator, congratulations! There's no reason to harsh your high because there's nothing wrong with it. Vibrators are excellent tools to help you reach orgasm, particularly when it feels challenging or unobtainable.

If you're concerned about becoming too accustomed to your new sex toy, try approaching this with balance in mind. Masturbate with your sex toy one day and then masturbate with your hands the next. Use your vibrator during a sexual experience with your partner and then try having sex without it another time. If you don't orgasm but really want to, then shamelessly bust out that vibrator during or after your sexy-time sessions because pleasure is your birthright.

If you can only orgasm with a vibrator, and you feel like this is a problem for you because *you* want to learn how to orgasm in other ways, just take a break from your sex toy. Take thirty days off from using your vibe and drop into each of your pleasure experiences using hands, mouths, or your mind. Although it will take some time, your body and brain will begin to reprogram eventually, leading you to O Town in new ways. Be patient with yourself and remember that old saying: "It's not about the destination, it's about the journey."

Uncover Your Core Erotic Themes

It's time to bring partners into the equation. One way to uncover more about your unique turn-ons in a partnered setting is simply to ask yourself, *How do I want to feel during sex and intimacy?* Deeply consider the answer. Most people want to experience a particular feeling when they are in an erotic space. In his book *The Erotic Mind: Unlocking the Inner Sources of Passion and Fulfillment*, Jack Morin, PhD, refers to this as a "core erotic theme." Your core erotic themes are what you need to *feel* connected and be sexually engaged. It's your personal sexual wiring, and it's based on what makes you feel sexually alive. It's less about *what* you do sexually than *how* you want to *feel*. Being aware of your core erotic themes involves knowing what you want and need during sexual encounters and can help you be fully present as you explore them.

April knows that she wants to feel special and be told how she's unique, amazing, incredible, and the sexiest apple of her lover's eyes. On the other hand, Amy wants to feel cared for and brought to a place of respect, adoration, and safety where she can trust her partner to handle all aspects of her wild sexuality. Another common theme involves a desire to feel "the best" (best lover, the finest cock, most amazing pussy, best ass, etc.) that your partner has ever experienced. Other themes include feeling worshiped, precious, possessed, dominated, sacred, and so on. The way you identify with your core erotic theme is entirely defined by you.

 Unearth your own core erotic theme with episode #2, "How to Ask for What You Want (in the Bedroom)."

I'M NOT SURE WHAT SHOULD STAY FANTASY VERSUS REALITY IN MY SEX LIFE

I get turned on by the idea of having threesomes with all genders, doing kinky things, and anal play, but my partner is not open to any of it. I've been afraid to share this in past relationships, so I've never tried it out, but I'm unsure of what I actually want to do and what should remain fantasy. I want to honor my partner's needs, but I'm fearful I'll miss out on great sex. Is this valid or am I just delusional?

This question is multilayered. Some of those layers relate to mismatched and conflicting desires within long-term relationships, which we'll go over in Chapter 5. But the core of this question revolves around navigating the complex world of fantasies, especially when there is a desire for sexual variety and newness, things that prove to be key pieces to maintaining a sexually charged long-term relationship.

There's Nothing Wrong with Wanting Newness

Esther Perel, relationship expert, psychotherapist, and author of *Mating in Captivity* and *The State of Affairs*, has spent decades researching the common challenges of long-term partnerships, domesticity, and intimacy. Perel also happens to be *Shameless Sex*'s biggest (platonic) crush ever! Perel's years of work explore the concept of "newness" by breaking love down into two parts: surrender and autonomy, or the needs for togetherness and separateness, which exist alongside each other in any relationship. (Paradoxically, separateness is a precondition for connection.)

Perel shares a simple equation to further illuminate this complexity: Attraction + Obstacle = Desire. In this equation, attraction refers to being attracted to a person's looks, intellect, personality, social status, other attributes, or all of the above. Obstacle equates to some kind of newness—such as that feeling of mystery that occurs in the beginning of a relationship, prior to the point when the connection enters the secure "you're mine" stage.

Before breaking open the results of this desire equation, let's remember that people are not property, and while you may feel comfortable in the relationship because you "put a ring on it" or you live together and have assets and children, your partner is their own person, and you can't own people. They do not belong to you and are not yours for the keeping, nor are you fully safe from losing the relationship just because you feel secure at this point in time. It's obvious and unfortunate that there are relationships where partners (predominantly women) do not have the right nor the safety to leave even if they desire. In the world today, there are millions of humans who either lack the ability to feel or to exercise their sexual and relational autonomy. Hopefully, this is something that's changing because everyone deserves the freedom to choose the partners and the pleasure they deserve. But for the privileged people who do have the choice: Every day is a new opportunity with your partner(s). Just because things feel "okay," "fine," or "good enough," and you're "fairly happy," it's important to recognize the possibility that your partner may not be yours forever.

Let's face it: Desire isn't easy to wrap your head around. It can seem selfish and even inappropriate (gasp!). But it also can make or break a partnership. Most humans will crave adventure at some point in their long-term relationships, even while they feel a deep sense of love and fulfillment. This craving for newness is because love and desire thrive in very different situations. While love grows when you feel strongly bonded and connected to another person, desire is the yearning for the unpredictable—that "butterflies in your stomach" excitement. When a partnership becomes predictable and the mystery leaves, it's usually because love has created security and safety, making you comfortable. And, although comfort is nice, it can be a desire killer if it's not seasoned with a little newness every now and then.

Dr. Christopher Ryan, co-author of *Sex at Dawn: How We Mate, Why We Stray, and What It Means for Modern Relationships*, and Wednesday Martin, PhD, agree there is nothing unusual about desiring something beyond your everyday intimate experiences. No matter what you're into or how you identify, the desire for variety and newness is more common than society would have you believe.

 Uncover the truth about having desire for others in episode #32, "Masturbation, How to Be an Authentic Lover, & Sex at Dawn—with Dr. Christopher Ryan."

Desire Discrepancies

Desire is about the excitement you crave, want, or yearn for. It's a range of feelings and things that can turn you on and be unfamiliar, naughty, playful, and even raunchy. If you feel like you don't have desire but you long for it, then it may be something you wish to receive from your partner(s). As Esther Perel's work suggests, desire is often easy during the beginning of a relationship—there's a reason it's known as the "lust" or "honeymoon" phase. But don't get it twisted: Just because novelty wears off and desire shifts and sometimes fades away doesn't mean your relationship has to be over. Differences in desire between partners, also known as a "desire discrepancy," are somewhat unavoidable in long-term relationships, but it doesn't have to be a problem and there are ways to get desire back.

However, while desire discrepancies are definitely workable, discrepancies in core values (about relationships or the world) are a bit more significant. If you find yourself in a place where your core values, including (but not limited to) sex, emotional connection, parenting, health, family, procreation, finances, politics, or human rights are not in alignment with that of your partner, then this could be worthy of serious consideration. Before making any assumptions (because to ASSUME is to make an ASS out of U and ME), let's look at the possible Pleasure Paths so you can choose which way to go.

I'M NOT SURE WHAT SHOULD STAY FANTASY VERSUS REALITY IN MY SEX LIFE

1. Would you like to learn how to uncover and explore your fantasies? If so, continue to read this chapter.

2. Do you want to discover how to share your desires beyond what you've attempted before? Do you want to be able to add more ease to this conversation, learn to advocate for your desires, and refine the art of sexual negotiation? If so, continue to read this chapter. Also, go to page **148** of **Chapter 4: How Can I Ask for What I Want or Even Talk About Sex?** for the CONNECT formula, which will help you navigate these tricky conversations.

3. Are you in a place where you've tried to express your desires, yet your partner is a hard no on certain things that are feeling like an undeniable part of you? Are you questioning the compatibility of the relationship, feeling like you have mismatched desires, or considering asking for some form of nonmonogamy? If so, continue reading this chapter. Also, go to page **168** of **Chapter 5: Are We Broken?** for additional tools to apply if any of these complex relationship scenarios are at play.

Fantasy Versus Desire

Both Amy and April have firsthand experience with the distinction between sexual fantasy and reality. Some material is meant to reside in the internal spank bank (the thoughts that get your juices flowing)—just because it's a fantasy doesn't mean you want to act it out in real life. Amy has been turned on by coercive sex fantasies since well before she became sexually active. While she's experienced a fair amount of coercive sexual experiences, none resembled her fantasy, and she has no desire to repeat them. Even so, these thoughts still get her pussy juices flowing.

April's stepparent fantasy is similar. April has never had any desire to have sex with an actual stepparent, but she's still turned on by the idea of submission to a power role, as in a daddy/stepdaughter, professor/student, or boss/employee dynamic. These types of power relinquishments are arousing for her because she's a person who is in control of most things outside of the bedroom, so the thought of having sex with a person of authority who's telling her what to do is taboo, naughty, and gets her horny every time.

Dr. Justin Lehmiller, fantasy and sexuality expert and author of *Tell Me What You Want: The Science of Sexual Desire and How It Can Help You Improve Your Sex Life* shares a brilliant insight on fantasy: "There's a difference between a sexual *fantasy* and a sexual *desire*. A fantasy is simply a mental picture that is sexually arousing to you; it doesn't necessarily have to be something you want to do. On the other hand, a desire is something you truly want to experience. Your fantasies could be desires, but they don't have to be. . . Sometimes a fantasy is just a fantasy. Even though we may know there's no possibility of it happening or we don't want it to materialize, it's the idea of it which turns us on for some reason, whether it's a result of cultural conditioning factors or just a spontaneous thought that pops into your head and gets you aroused. We don't always know how to explain it, but sometimes a thought just turns us on, even though we have no desire to actually experience it in real life."

Exploring her sexual imagination, when she felt safe enough with someone, has helped April shake up her bedroom routine and promote excitement in her long-term relationship. After months of hesitation for fear that it would lead to insecurities that could strain their relationship, she finally shared her fantasy of shagging a British taxicab driver with her partner. She explained that she didn't want to act it out in real life but thought it was totally hot and completely obscene. Instead of getting pushback, she was surprised when her partner said out of the blue a few nights later, "Your ride is here" in his best British accent. He led her to the bedroom, where they pretended the bed was the back of the cab and sucking and fucking was the fare she had to pay. Not only was it extremely sexy, but it created a new sense of connection in their relationship that was followed by even more desire for each other.

As Dr. Lehmiller's research demonstrates, the world of fantasy is endless and individually unique, and there is nothing wrong with what turns you on within your own mind. It can also help you uncover the desires you want to bring to life. Dr. Lehmiller finds in his research that "what people describe as their favorite all-time fantasy does tend to be a desire more often than not. It's usually something they want to act out and make a part of their sexual reality. However, it's important to note that your favorite fantasy is typically just one of many. People can have hundreds, even thousands, of fantasies over the course of their lives and they don't necessarily want to act on all of them."

Time to fantasize about your fantasies. What is your ultimate fantasy—the one that you crave to bring into fruition? What is your go-to spank bank material? What do these scenes, actions, and behaviors entail? How long have you had these fantasies? What comes up for you when you imagine yourself with complete freedom to explore these fantasies with consenting people you're sexually attracted to? Envision a world where your partner is a big yes and now anything is on the table. What feelings come up as you visualize yourself acting out these scenarios?

If you have a clear understanding of your ultimate fantasy, and that fantasy has been with you for quite some time and brings you positive feelings (like arousal, excitement, aliveness, and maybe even some nervousness) when you imagine it happening, then this is something you may be meant to explore in real life (as long as it's consensual, of course!). But now what do you do if your partner isn't interested in helping you act out your fantasies?

If you've shared your fantasies with your partner, but they've told you, "No, it's not my thing," consider what it would be like to redo this conversation once you have a bit more clarity. Assess the options and see if there are ways you two can work together to find a mutually pleasurable solution. Dr. Lehmiller recommends starting low and slow when sharing your fantasies. He says, "Don't jump into the kinkiest thing you can possibly think of. Start with something tamer, and as you share your fantasies, validate your partner. Tell them how they play an important and central role in your fantasy and how this isn't about you wanting to get rid of them or replace them and how much you enjoy the sex you're already having together."

According to Dr. Lehmiller, it is likely that your partner will be more receptive to the idea if they feel validated and if you present it as a means of adding something new to your shared sex life, with the intention of maximizing pleasure for everyone. He explains, "All of these things are ways that you can potentially start these conversations—and then, eventually, move down the path of sharing your more adventurous fantasies, and maybe even acting on some of them as well, so long as you prioritize mutual consent, safety, and pleasure along the way."

However, it requires a considerate approach and a safe environment. As Dr. Lehmiller puts it, "When it comes to that first hurdle of sharing your fantasies with your partner, you need to start by making sure you feel good about yourself and what you're fantasizing about so that shame doesn't hold you back. Then choose the right time and place to have a discussion about sexual fantasies. Ideally, you want to do this in a quiet, private place." It's also crucial to have this conversation outside of sexy time. Taking the time to discuss this outside of a sexual context will help offset any potential hurt or confusion and allow everyone to focus on the dialogue.

If you're considering introducing new sexual practices into your relationship, how did you convey your fantasies in the past? What was the environment like? Are you seeing an opportunity to try again while applying the new tools you are learning? This is *not* an invitation to implement any form of nonconsensual manipulation or coercion. Instead, think about the ways you've already attemped to share you desires. There is a possibility your partner didn't hear how important these aspects were to you in the first place, and they may be afraid of what might happen if you start exploring these fantasies. Maybe your partner has fantasies too, but they're trapped in a cage of shame, thinking something is wrong with the stimulating thoughts in their own spank bank. But if you feel that you've shared what's on your mind and your partner still says no, then don't push them. There are various ways to approach mismatched desires if they become a problem in your relationship, and you can check those out in Chapter 5.

 Learn more about the science behind fantasy in episode #98, "The Science of Sexual Fantasy—with Dr. Justin Lehmiller."

Implementing Fantasy in Real Life (Or Not)

As trauma-informed intimacy coach and educator Dr. Alison Ash's work underscores, feeling disconnected from one's own fantasies is very normal. According to Dr. Ash, "Some people feel like it's hard to have sexual fantasies, and what I often ask them is: 'Have you ever thought about what you would do with a million dollars? Or what your ideal date would be? Or your favorite vacation?', with the intention of helping them realize that their ability to fantasize is more accessible than they thought." Beyond the accessibility of fantasies, Dr. Ash also emphasizes their benefits. She continues, "[Fantasizing is] a wonderful place to start to explore your desires with utter permission. I really like to emphasize the mental liberation component of fantasizing, that you have the right to think about whatever you want to. You can have fantasies that you never want to have happen in real life."

Dr. Ash's words highlight that getting curious about your partner's fantasies can have positive effects on your sex life—at least, in the right setting, which you'll learn more about in a moment. Do they have any fantasies that turn them on, even if they're things they don't want to materialize in real life? Have they ever used their imagination to heighten their arousal, and if so, what scenarios were they playing with? Cultivate your curiosity through gentle communication and within a safe context, and you might find there's much more to your partner's sexuality than you think.

Even if your partner is open to discussing fantasies (and maybe even exploring some of them), you may still need to negotiate. When negotiating, Dr. Ash emphasizes working together in a way that takes everyone's needs into account. In her words, conversations like these "may be an opportunity to create a fantasy together . . .Whether you are sharing fantasies with a person or you're enacting a role-play situation, consent is absolutely necessary. If you're going to share a fantasy, ask permission first: 'I'd love to share a fantasy with you. Are you open to hearing it?' If at any point someone wants to stop, that is their right. The next question may be, 'Would you like to role-play or to create this fantasy together?'" Dr. Ash brings up some very important points about the right situations in which to discuss fantasies. These are the key factors to consider when it comes to bringing fantasty to fruition: aka the "Three Cs."

Three Cs of Fantasy: Consent, Curiosity, and Co-Creation

If your partner is open to exploring your fantasies, make sure the Three Cs are present. *Consent* requires all parties to be a full, active fuck yes. *Curiosity* is about taking the time to understand and consider everyone's needs and desires. *Co-creation* entails putting the puzzle pieces together to produce a sexual experience that feels good for everyone. With all Three Cs in place, magic may ensue.

Amy was able to implement her fantasies by exploring dominance, submission, and role-play. When her partner consented and maintained curiosity about her desires, she acted out being a "dirty little slut" and "naughty little schoolgirl" within a safe container of play. She's also pretended to be a sex worker named Cali who gets paid by her "client" (a partner) to provide a sexual experience that Cali chooses—because she paid her way through medical school and is empowered to fuck however she pleases. Some of Amy's partners were not interested in co-creating this form of sexual experience with her, which was 100 percent their right to choose. It's also a point where these partners' sexual needs became less compatible with hers, which was okay too.

As Dr. Alison Ash emphasizes, "No matter what you do, get consent every step of the way." She continues, "Let's say that I'm a yes to role-playing a threesome, but not a yes to doing it with an actual person. In this case, we may dirty talk a threesome scenario or use a sex toy as the stand-in for the third person—or maybe my partner leaves the room and comes back using a different voice, and we pretend it's a new person. . . If we decide we want to actually have a threesome in real life, this would involve getting consent with my partner and the third person, where we all talk about what we do and don't want to experience together. If all parties are unable to consent to the act of sharing fantasies, creating a role-play scenario, or the actual enactment of it in real life, perhaps it should just stay in your fantasy mind."

Think of consent as a paintbrush on your erotic canvas. Without it, you can only create a messy finger-painted portrait that your own parents wouldn't even frame. But when painting with the polished paintbrush of consent, a beautiful masterpiece may follow—one that can hang on the wall for everyone to enjoy.

Dr. Ash also gives various examples of ways partners can lean into each other, even if it doesn't mean fulfilling the ultimate fantasy to a T. This is where *curiosity* and *co-creation* come in. From threesomes to anal play to kink and beyond, there are many options on the table to add to your *yes* and *maybe* lists for sexual exploration, but they require a lot of discussion and working together. This is not the same as complying or tolerating. It's when two or more parties share and listen to each other's desires and boundaries, and then get creative about how they can meet somewhere close to the middle, where everyone feels good and everyone's needs are accounted for.

 Discover new ways to play into your erotic fantasies in episode #253, "Keeping It Hot with Fantasies and Role-Play—with Dr. Alison Ash."

Sex Outside Your Orientation Box

You may desire to explore sex with people beyond what you think of as your preferred gender(s)—and this is completely normal. For some, this can be a stepping stone toward realizing their orientation is different than they thought it was. But just because you feel this way does not mean you need to change your label, or even pick one at all. You are the only person who can label you. It can also be helpful to keep in mind that labels are fluid and can change at any time—no matter what you choose, you're not signing anything in blood.

Amy's mom, Janis, identified as a straight cis woman until her fifties. If you asked her how she felt about the idea of having sex with another woman before then, she would have said, "It's something I'm not opposed to, but I've never had the opportunity to explore it." Well, that opportunity finally came, and she was able to realize that she's more bisexual than straight. She sometimes uses the term "queer" to refer to her orientation, but most of the time, she prefers not to take on any labels at all.

> We thought at least one "your mom" joke was necessary:
>
> Knock knock!
>
> *Who's there?*
>
> Your mom.
>
> *Your mom who?*
>
> Your mom who's queer, has no fear, and says labels are for food!

Orientation Identity Versus Fantasy Within a Relationship

As is true of all fantasies, whether you choose to seek intimacy outside of your usual preferred gender(s) is up to you. Only you can decide if a fantasy is meant to be acted out in real life or not. If this desire feels important and like something you need in reality, then consider the safe and fulfilling ways you could explore them. What if you paid a sex worker for webcam sex? And if this is the direction you choose, then how does your partner feel about it? That's when you dust off your respectful negotiation skills. Maybe they're a yes, but they'd like to be present while you're having cam sex, or maybe they're a no to being present but feel safe enough for you to explore it on your own. Discuss specifics: Do the sexual interactions need to involve viewing (voyeurism), exhibiting (exhibitionism), or genitals and penetration, or is it about the words shared and having intimate connection? Through open communication, as well as plenty of negotiation, you might be surprised at how many options are available to try and create a win-win within your relationship.

A person's sexual identity, including their orientation, is an innate part of themselves. It's not something that can be suddenly changed or removed from their system. Remember, you can't "pray the gay away" (nor should you, because you were designed to be exactly as you are—beautifully unique and irreplaceable!). If you're abiding by consent, there is nothing you need to change about your identity or deep desires to appease any relationship or social norms. And if these desires feel like an intrinsic part of you, yet they still go unmet, you will likely continue to experience dissatisfaction and distress.

GET THAT BIG D (DESIRE!)

While sexuality will vary from person to person and shift throughout a lifetime, everyone has sexual desires that reflect their unique selves. Yet, beyond being able to recognize your desires, you may struggle to experience the full pleasure that they bring if you don't get clear on what they entail. Whether you're just getting to know your erotic self or are navigating a challenging relationship that seems to be shutting your desire door, there are lots of things you can do to get in touch with that big D again.

As you take the journey to reclaim your sexual self and find the freedom to express your core desires, use the tools in this chapter to help you along the way. And remember, it's okay to break the rules sometimes—or at least to be open to the possibility that you might not do things perfectly. When you've got boundaries (and consent), you have room for experimenting and exploring what feels good for you, without feeling bad about it if those fantasies don't end up being as sexy as you imagined they would be. And don't be scared to try something that feels slightly out of your comfort zone because the novelty just might fire up that big D and ignite the passion in your relationship.

Lastly, when it comes to long-term relationships, the best way to explore your erotic world is with someone who values you and is willing to go along with you on the ride. Even better if they make it their ride too! Allow yourself to try new things and invite your partner to have conversations about what they're craving sexually as well. If you're feeling a bit overwhelmed about how to discuss your desires, look no further for help than the next chapter, which is all about how to ask for what you want and need in the bedroom. Are you ready to become a pro at sexual and relational communication? Then turn the page and read on.

How Can I Ask for What I Want or Even Talk About Sex?

This chapter centers around perhaps the most foundational part of sex and relationships: communication. Even if you're an amazing communicator in other aspects of your life, expressing your sexual desires and talking about them can be really tough—sometimes even *we* struggle with talking about sex, and it's our specialty. But have no fear: after reading this chapter, you'll be able to advocate for yourself like a pro.

In the previous chapter, you became an archaeologist of yourself by digging deep to uncover and understand your sexual desires. Now, it's time to learn how to share your discoveries with your partner(s). The following pages will focus on the actual relational part of communication and how to break any patterns of putting your desires on the back burner when sharing intimately with a partner.

TALKING ABOUT SEX IS HARD!

There are countless reasons you might ignore your own needs or feel a tinge of terror when talking about sex. Shame, trauma, gender expectations, and people-pleasing are just a few that we've covered in Chapters 2 and 3. All of these experiences factor into your level of comfort when talking about sex. For many people, this discomfort stems from a lack of education around sexual self-advocacy and the absence of positive examples of how to speak with openness and honesty. There's an underlying notion in most cultures that talking about sex is shameful, taboo, and socially unacceptable.

These beliefs can linger in sexual environments or contexts as well. Most people wouldn't consider "toleration" and "compliance" to be sexy words (unless they're used in the world of consensual kink), and yet tolerating and complying are common within sex and relationships. It's tempting to just go with the flow and avoid speaking up about what you want, especially when there's fear of rejection, abandonment, feeling like you're doing something wrong, or that you're "killing the mood." These fears frequently date back to the limiting beliefs you developed from your childhood experiences. The path to having more empowering sexual experiences requires the combination of healing from the past and practicing the expression of your sexual needs.

Amy can deeply relate to these fears. Her first time touching a penis was also one of her first experiences with feeling disempowered. She was thirteen and among a group of people at a friend's house—including her friend's older brother, who sometimes bullied Amy. In a dark room, her friend's brother asked Amy to give him a massage on his back, and then his stomach. He proceeded to push her hand down toward his penis and then used his hand over hers to jerk himself off until he finished. She did not know how to pull her hand away and say, "I do not want to do this" because she was afraid of how he might respond to her. So, she tolerated the experience, but she felt terrible afterward. For a long time, that experience shaped how Amy viewed herself when getting intimate with others. Only after years of work can Amy now finally advocate for herself and her body knowing she does not get touched, nor will she give touch, without full and active consent—a process that often involves deep conversation and negotiation.

Healing from these limiting beliefs involves introspection into what, why, and how they developed in the first place. Think about these important questions: *What life experiences contributed to your fear of speaking up for yourself? Why do you quiet your voice? How has this silence protected you? Has this prevented you from living as your best self and if so, in what ways? What do you truly need or desire sexually?* If you find the answers to these questions emotionally triggering, then this may be the time to work on renewing these pieces with the guidance of a therapist or coach. As expressed before, a trip into the past can stir up some unresolved pain and emotional wounds. This pain deserves your attention, and having the support of a trained professional can make this process easier and prevent overwhelm and re-traumatization.

After you have more clarity on the reasons behind your fears and limiting beliefs around sexual self-advocacy, then you can move to the practice phase of this learning process. The good news is that this can be enjoyable, playful, and sometimes even arousing. There are even techniques that can help you transform talking about sex and desire into a playful and flirtatious game of negotiation rather than a terrifying period of raw vulnerability.

However, practice takes time, patience, and can be risky (especially while maintaining your boundaries). If you're a beginner to asking for what you want or talking about sex, it's natural for it to feel uncomfortable, awkward, tiresome, and a little scary. But never fear, *Shameless Sex* is here! Even Olympic athletes need coaches, and we'll make this "training" easier by starting you off with basic tips and drills you can practice. And just like an athlete, the more you practice, the more strength and confidence you'll build—furthering your potential for sexual glory (and maybe even a gold medal in communication).

I DON'T KNOW HOW TO TALK ABOUT TRYING NEW THINGS WITH MY PARTNER

I'm open to my sexuality more than ever before since listening to your podcast. My sex drive is through the roof! But I'm in a relationship with a partner who has a hard time sharing anything about sexual desires. I've tried to initiate these types of conversations, but my effort has never been reciprocated. In the past, I would have pushed my feelings down, but that's not an option anymore because I now know what I want in the bedroom. How do I tell my partner I want more foreplay, sex, newness, positions, and touch without leading to a defensive shutdown?

It's not unusual to have a mismatch in communication abilities around sex and desire, and it can happen with both casual sex and committed relationships. Previous experiences and prior conditioning affect how each individual communicates about sex. This is important to understand because it means that each person is only capable of showing up based on where they stand at that given time.

April can recount several past relationships where she felt frustration due to the differing or, worse yet, downright poor communication styles of her sexual partners. One partner, now called the "master of defense," would shift blame whenever he felt threatened or insecure in a conversation, denying anything he considered a criticism and insinuating that April's thinking was irrational if it wasn't in line with his. Another, now known as the "prince of procrastination," would insist, time and again, that he was committed to doing the work to improve their intimacy issues. April would see him browsing books on healthy communication and hear him making promises about going to therapy sessions, but he never followed through with any of it. Year after year, the same sex and intimacy issues would arise until the relationship dissolved. We wouldn't wish such circumstances on anyone, because our goal is to see you thrive. But luckily, we have some helpful recommendations for fostering genuine openness in sexual and relational communication.

Even if you're in an established relationship, these communication tips can still be crucial. Many people only come into their sexual power after they've invested time and effort into a long-term partnership. While each partner presumably entered the relationship with similar perspectives, they may reach roadblocks to compatibility as they each continue to better understand their own needs. If you are in a relationship where you recognize your dissatisfaction and appreciate the importance of speaking to your needs and desires, get ready because this chapter has a ton of applicable tools for you.

Talking About "Talking About Sex"

Talking about "talking about sex" sounds like a mindfuck, so here is a comparison you can (hopefully) relate to. You bring your car to a mechanic, and they begin discussing the ways they can work on your vehicle. While they're telling you about the parts they need to fix, you realize you have no idea what they are talking about. It sounds like another language. "That catalytic converter makes your oil dry, your flux capacitor is broken, your bushes on the wishbone are going, and you top off these fluids so you can have the ultimate performance . . ." Huh, say what!? This kind of shoptalk, especially if you have no practice with the language, can be intimidating and confusing. Similarly, articulating sexual wants and needs if you have little to no experience can be daunting. How are you going to understand, drop in, and feel comfortable expressing yourself further if you haven't prepared beforehand? You need to feel a level of confidence and security before discussing the X, Y, and Z of what you want so you can effectively address the issues at hand.

 Perfect the art of "talking about talking about sex" in episode #162, "What Do I Want and How Do I Ask for It—with Monica Jayne."

Navigating communication breakdowns in partnerships can be an art form, with entire books dedicated to the topic. Two books that have been instrumental in improving April's communication skills are *Taking the War Out of Our Words: The Art of Powerful Non-Defensive Communication* by Sharon Strand Ellison and *Nonviolent Communication: A Language of Life* by Marshall B. Rosenberg, PhD. By learning nonviolent communication skills, you can build integrity, eliminate defensiveness, and promote kindness in your relationships. These techniques are powerful enough to transform your life by turning conflicts into cooperation. Fortunately, you can acquire a solid foundation in these methods by reading this book, so keep turning the page to find out which Pleasure Path suits you best. Trust us, it's worth your while.

I DON'T KNOW HOW TO TALK ABOUT TRYING NEW THINGS WITH MY PARTNER

1. Do you want to develop the skills necessary for talking about sex? Would you like to share the importance of being in a partnership where you can express your sexual wants and engage in discussions with your partner about their desires too? If so, continue to read this chapter.

2. Are you interested in a framework for having these difficult conversations in a way that's less likely to trigger defensiveness in your partner? Or are you already feeling skilled at having these conversations, but would like to refine your approach even further? If so, continue to read this chapter.

3. Do you feel like you've tried everything possible to express your needs, yet you continue to find yourself in a place where nothing has changed? If so, it may be time to consider reframing the relationship. To learn more, go to page **174** of **Chapter 5: Are We Broken?** for ways to reformat your relationship so it can better serve you.

Permission and Big Versus Small Asks

Broaching these potentially intense topics requires permission from the other person(s). No, that doesn't mean you need to get down on your knees and ask your partner for their approval to bring up a potentially heated subject (unless this is part of a pre-negotiated BDSM role-play game—then by all means, get down and beg!). Instead, remember that everyone involved needs to feel prioritized and respected. This includes considering the time, place, and emotional capacity of each person before initiating any potentially triggering or stressful conversations about sex and relationships.

Let's simplify things and divide these interactions into two general categories: *Small Asks* and *Big Asks*. A Small Ask is when you voice something that feels light yet slightly uncomfortable, usually a small request to adjust something that is already occurring. Examples of Small Asks would be requesting for your partner to try a different tone when speaking to you or asking if they can touch your body in a different way. A Big Ask could potentially bring up strong emotions and lead to longer discussions. Examples of Big Asks include sharing your hurt about how you feel your partner is (or isn't) showing up for you or addressing your desire for a major shift in the way you engage sexually. No matter the interaction, try using language that's loving and considerate. This can turn a Small Ask into an instantaneous resolution and also helps to lessen the reactionary potential of a Big Ask, which generally requires more time, care, and attention. Keep in mind, what seems like a Small Ask to you might be a Big Ask to your partner. Therefore, it's wise to avoid expectations and be prepared to handle any strong emotions that may arise during the process.

Small Asks

Think of Small Asks as adjustments to something you would prefer be done differently. Try this three-step formula: 1) Start with an authentic compliment or praise; 2) follow it with "AND," not "but"; and 3) make the request for what you want. Unlike Big Asks, Small Asks can be made in the heat of the moment when bodies are already interacting in an intimate way.

Role-play time: Imagine your partner is massaging your back. While it feels nice to receive touch from them, they continuously rub and knead the same spot to the point where it's irritating your skin. Your mind is weighing the options: tolerating the touch to keep the peace or speaking what you truly desire. If you choose the first option, not only could the irritation pull you out of being present (possibly leading to a missed opportunity for deep connection), but you're enabling a behavior that doesn't work for you—which means it could happen again. If you choose the second option, you increase your chances of receiving what you want, while risking a breach in connection if your partner doesn't respond well to your request.

If you'd like to express your truth in a way that decreases the risk of losing affection, you can say something like *I love when you massage my back, AND what I'd love even more is if you'd use longer strokes all over my entire back and down my legs too*. With the right context and tone, many people will hear this direction as a compliment rather than a criticism and will happily follow through with the request you just made. Also, keep in mind that a request is *not* a demand, and your partner may have boundaries around your requests, which is totally acceptable.

Big Asks

Big Asks require more consideration, intention, and time. Big Asks generally work best when all parties are not in a hurry or distracted, are in good spirits, are given the opportunity to grant their own autonomous permission to enter the dialogue, and are in a private space outside of sexy time. For example, a Big Ask could involve the need to receive touch from your partner via their hands and mouth. It could even be a "Big Ask 2.0" if it's a request you've brought up before but you're now advocating for it with greater awareness of its importance. Your desire to receive touch from your partner in a way that's mutually reciprocated is essential.

We understand that Big Asks can be stressful, and it's hard to know the best way to approach them. That's why we've condensed our most valuable tips on the subject into a formula called CONNECT, because we want to make sure this process is as painless (and productive) as possible.

CONNECT

When it comes to initiating more complicated conversations with your partner about sex and relationships, CONNECT is here to help. Maybe you've already tried sharing your wants and needs but to no avail—or perhaps this is your first attempt at having this type of dialogue. Either way, you can count on CONNECT. If your partner is resistant to opening up, and you're met with barriers due to fear, shame, or conditioning, don't worry—these seven clever strategies can help you navigate challenging conversations about sex and intimacy.

CONNECT: Seven *Shameless Sex* Strategies for Having Difficult Conversations Around Sex

1. **Consideration.** Be considerate and approach the topic when both you and your partner are in good spirits. Timing can be everything, so do your best to avoid potential low energetic periods such as entering or exiting a stressful day. Open the conversation when each person seems to be in a positive mindset and has the energy to listen.

2. **Outside.** Have the discussion outside of the bedroom and as far away from any sexual activity as possible. If you're still naked or just finished having sex, this is *not* the ideal time to approach the subject. Sleep on it and address the topic when you're both out of a sexual space.

3. **Negotiation.** Ask for permission to share and negotiate the terms of the conversation based on your mutual needs. Instead of cornering your partner, let them know there's something important coming up for you about your relationship and ask if now is a good time to talk about it. If you get a no, invite them to share what time would be good for them. You can assert yourself and lovingly suggest a time (tomorrow over coffee, lunch on Wednesday, after we put the kids to bed tonight, etc.). However, while it's beneficial to have a set time, it's still important to check in again just beforehand.

   Here's a broad script you can reference to help initiate the conversation: *Hey lovie, there's something important coming up for me about our relationship. Is now a good time to talk? If not, I understand. How about we talk tomorrow at ____ o'clock instead? Let's check in beforehand to make sure it still feels like the right time. And*

I really need you to know how important this is to me, so I hope we can prioritize this conversation.

4. **Nicely to the nitty-gritty.** Start with the positives and be authentic. Open the conversation by sharing all the ways you value your partner and your relationship. Then move on to the aspects of sex and pleasure that are feeling good and in alignment for you. This is not about manipulating the conversation but instead is about being as real and kind as possible. Yes, you have an intention of getting something out of this discussion, but it's also an opportunity to remind your partner that you care and to applaud the aspects of the relationship that you're grateful for. Remember to press pause and request more time to gather your thoughts if the conversation gets too heated or hurtful, or if your inner people pleaser starts emerging and you steer away from addressing your needs to avoid further conflict.

5. **Exposure.** Be willing to be vulnerable. This is the time to expose your inner erotic landscape, and that's not easy—in fact, it will take a significant amount of courage, honesty, and personal ownership of who you are. To get the most out of this conversation, sit down beforehand and write out all the ways you may have contributed to the disconnection you're feeling. What are some of the things you could have done better? Also, be considerate of your partner's experience before and during this conversation. Remember the reasons you're initiating the conversation: not because your partner isn't good enough or there's something wrong with them, but because you want to work on improving communication in a partnership that's important to you (and ultimately enhance your relationship).

6. **Curiosity.** Get curious about what your partner is feeling or experiencing. Make this conversation more about "we" and less about "me" or "you." Instead of pointing fingers and saying, "You do too much of this and not enough of that" or, "You're always doing this and never doing that," flip the script instead: "I want this for us. I want to go from okay to good or from good to great in a way that makes us more connected sexually and emotionally than ever before." In other words, you're inviting your partner to lean into you while you're simultaneously leaning into them.

7. **Therapy.** Seek a therapist or coach. If you're hitting a wall in your relationship and feeling stuck, triggered, or spinning in circles, it's time to consider working with a professional. Advocating for this means standing firm on the importance of seeking outside support without coercing or pushing in a way that feels forceful. Again, make it an "us" or "we" exchange by saying something like, "We're stuck here, and our relationship is important to me. I would love it if we could explore some outside help so we can get more tools from an unbiased third party. Are you open to looking for someone together?" Ultimately, finding a professional you both feel comfortable and safe with is essential and will help you move forward.

Prompts for CONNECTing

Let's say you implement the first three steps of CONNECT and your partner is open to having this conversation. What's next? Here are some ways to kick off the conversation:

- **Start with the positives.** "I really appreciate you taking the time to listen to me. I love you and I'm excited to deepen our relationship." Or, "To me, part of going deeper in our relationship is being able to talk to you about sex and what we each want and fantasize about."

- **Be vulnerable and honest.** "It's really important for me to be able to talk about sex with you. I want to share my sexual needs, and I want to hear your needs too so I can better understand you."

- **Take accountablility for your role.** "Communicating like this is new to me because I've spent my life putting my own sexual needs to the side. I know this is confusing because I've done that in this relationship too, but I don't want to do that anymore."

- **Be curious and avoid blame.** "I feel like I've shared my desires in the past but never got to hear about yours. What is your experience around that? Are you open to us sharing our desires? Would you be into creating a sexual menu together to define our yeses, nos, and maybes?"

Unfortunately, there are no guarantees your partner won't shut down or get defensive. After all, they're an individual with their own stuff. There's no magic formula to make everyone feel a specific way—nor is it your job to take that on. However, if you navigate the conversation with love, gentleness, accountability, authenticity, and curiosity, you will most likely be met with the same ease and openness in return. No matter how your partner responds, try listening to each word while empathizing with their experience. Give them space to speak—or to be silent, if that's what they need to collect their thoughts. If one or both of you tend to interrupt or talk over the other, designate an object as a "talking stick" and agree that only the person holding the talking stick can speak, while the other person *actively* listens. Switch off every few minutes or so. Use whichever method works best for you to create a space where both of you have the opportunity to speak and be heard equally, with the undivided attention of one another.

To ensure you're being heard, we also encourage you to steer the conversation away from a "tit for tat" approach. So instead of using a list of ways you pleasure your partner as ammunition to make your point, stick to advocating for your individual needs. You don't have to "earn" getting your needs met—and also, you're (hopefully) choosing to give pleasure because you want to, not because you're performing a duty or expecting something in return. In fact, using the "I do this for you so you should do this for me" line often ends up in a huge clusterfuck. Get clear with yourself: *What do you truly want and need? What are your boundaries and how far are you willing to lean in?* Speak to these key pieces lovingly while getting curious about your partner's unique perspective at the same time.

What Happens If You're Met with Resistance?

When someone resorts to blame, manipulation, gaslighting, interrogation, name-calling, or other forms of violent communication, it's a clear indication they are operating from a triggered or defensive space. It's important not to just tolerate this behavior. If possible, the calmer, less triggered person should suggest (or nonverbally signal) that it's the time to press pause on the conversation. Little can be done until everyone's system has calmed down. Your instinct may be to defend yourself or placate the other person's feelings, but the best tool to defuse the situation is to take a break from the conversation.

Taking a break does not mean shutting down or walking away without explanation. Instead, it's simply a matter of pulling a different tool out of your communication tool kit. If you're the one asking for the pause, convey your needs with loving reassurance. Be clear: State your intention for the pause and give an idea of how long you need to step away before you can revisit the discussion again. As Kate Loree, LMFT, explains, it's not helpful to leave another person hanging anxiously while one walks away indefinitely. This can feel hurtful for the anxious person and can create a bigger rupture in the relationship that will need its own new layer of repair later. If you're still unsure of how best to pause, consider including these three points:

- Give assurance and remove blame, making it a "we" thing instead of a "you" thing. For example: "I love you AND it feels like we're in a triggered state."
- Share your intention for the pause while also holding yourself accountable. For example: "I'm pressing pause right now because I need to recenter myself so I can speak from a calmer place."
- Share how long you'll be gone and your intention to continue to communicate, while still giving them autonomy. For example: "I'm going to go for a drive, and I'll be back in a few hours. If we're both feeling grounded when I come back AND if you're open to it, I would like to try to talk about it then. And if not, let's try to talk about it tomorrow."

> Develop more tools for tackling difficult conversations around sexuality in episode #283, "Building Loving Relationships, Nonmonogamy, and Attachment Styles— with Kate Loree, LMFT."

When you offer a time frame, do your best to follow through. Go for that drive—or whatever it is you need to do to take care of your nervous system in a supportive way—and come back at the time you proposed. Hopefully, your partner will take that time to care for themselves too, but this is out of your control. If you come back and they're still triggered, consider taking another, longer pause.

It's important to view the pause as an opportunity for negotiation as well. One person might desire to sleep on it while the other fears a sleepless night full of anxiety and needs some sort of resolution in the now. How can you approach your individual needs for space collectively? Before going to sleep, do you both have the capacity to reconnect with a hug and a few supportive words of love without returning to the disagreement at hand? Focus on granting space for the person who needs more time while providing reassurance for the one who wants immediate resolution.

Communicating with Casual Sex Partners

Communication is also crucial to the world of casual sexual relationships. Most people stumble through casual sex without solid communication techniques or practical ways of negotiating any needs and expectations with their partners. You have sex with someone once and it feels good, so you assume that it will continue to feel good when you have sex with them again. But what happens if connection deepens, or one person develops feelings while the other(s) wants to keep it casual? Consider the following casual hookup tips:

1. **Communicate.** Polish your communication skills. This is the perfect opportunity to practice speaking with transparency and self-advocacy. Research, study, and practice how to speak lovingly during difficult situations.

2. **Be honest.** If you know you're a hard no to exploring beyond the casual, share this from the beginning. Let your lover(s) know your current understanding about what is on and off the table. This does not mean you need to know exactly what the future holds, because things can change. It's about sharing what you know to be true for you in the present moment, including your thoughts on moving beyond casual sex. Withholding information (or sugarcoating it) can result in confusion and hurt feelings, but these can be avoided by being up front and honest before sexy time begins. This also gives your potential lover(s) the opportunity to check in with themselves to see if their needs align with your current boundaries. Think of your honesty as an act of service for everyone involved.

3. **Check in.** If your encounter isn't a one-off, initiate regular check-ins with your lover(s). Before reengaging in intimacy, share your thoughts and boundaries regarding the relational dynamic, and then inquire about theirs.

4. **Listen.** Even if you don't agree with what the other person wants, don't disregard their desires. Listen to them and get curious about their perspective. Their needs are just as valid as yours, and they deserve to be heard. Thank your lover(s) for their vulnerability by showing your support for their courage and emotional growth.

5. **Trust your gut.** Listen to your intuition. If your gut hints at the possibility of mismatched desires, check in with your lover(s) about it. A simple inquiry about how everyone is feeling can go a long way.

6. **Contemplate.** It's okay if you don't have the perfect words for expressing how you feel. If it gets confusing or ambiguous, speak to that. Say something like, "I've been enjoying spending time with you, and I have some feelings coming up right now; I need a few days to myself so I can better understand them."

7. **Create boundaries.** If you want to decrease the chances of people "catching feelings," consider establishing a boundary. You could, for example, set a rule that extensive cuddling and sleepovers are off the table because prolonged touch can create more oxytocin, a wonderful feel-good hormone related to attachment that can potentially build to deeper emotions. Share any boundaries that you have before entering an intimate space.

8. **Evaluate.** Note and evaluate how often you're seeing, calling, emailing, or messaging your lover(s). Because of those feel-good attachment hormones (as well as the stories the mind is so skilled at creating), regular engagement can increase the likelihood of attachment.

9. **Have respect.** Don't "ghost" people. If this is the exit route you usually take from sexual encounters, it's time to stop. It only creates

more confusion, hurt, and feelings of rejection when you suddenly "disappear" or stop engaging without warning. Instead, be a decent human (and not a total shit stain) and take the more considerate course of action by being honest about your desire to no longer see that person. It may seem daunting or feel like a hassle, but this person shared their body with you in some way, and the least you can do to honor that exchange is to be clear and up front with them.

 Become your most empowered, sex-positive, and slutty self by listening to episodes #5, "Casual Sex—with Reid Mihalko," and #206, "Getting It: A Guide to Hot, Healthy Hookups and Shame-Free Sex—with Allison Moon."

I WANT TO EXPLORE BDSM IN THE BEDROOM BUT I DON'T KNOW HOW TO ASK FOR IT

I'm in a relationship filled with great sex. The only thing missing is my desire to be dominated and experiment more with rough sex. It sounds so hot to be completely under my partner's control. We are really open with each other and I've shared my desire for BDSM, but it seems like the curiosity is combined with hesitation because my partner says they're "a lover and not a fighter." I don't want to add pressure, but this is something I really crave in the bedroom. How should I approach this so I can stay true to my desires while making sure my partner feels confident?

We know firsthand that it's totally normal to desire something that your partner feels hesitant about. Ten-year-old Amy discovered she had fantasies about being submissive after getting aroused by watching a sexually violent scene on *Melrose Place*. There was something about the idea of being dominated that felt really sexy to her. Fast-forward to age twenty, when she's in love and partnered for the first time. Though she knew nothing about kink or BDSM, she knew she wanted to bring these fantasies into real life. She tried to convey her desire to her partner by asking him to "make her feel small," but he was more confused than turned on by her request.

It wasn't until Amy entered the field of human sexuality that she learned about kink and BDSM. She finally understood how her request to "feel small" was an important desire she could identify as dominance and submission, and she also understood that not all lovers shared her same sexual craving or would be willing act on it.

In the words of sex educator and BDSM expert Midori, this type of erotic play is referred to as "a scene": a shared experience that is bounded by time, space, and consent, for the purpose of creating an arousing change of state. Creating a scene involves a lot of negotiation beforehand, as well as an idea of what might mutually entertain you in the moment. Sometimes, you won't want to engage in any form of kink or BDSM play—which makes it all the more necessary to have an expansive sexual menu that you check in with your partner(s) about regularly so you can identify what kinds of play all parties wish to engage in.

If, like Amy, your desire to explore dominance and submission resides beyond your spank bank, and you need to experience it in real life, sharing your desires and boundaries with your partner and working together to identify and express them is a critical first step.

Pre-Play Negotiation

Being hesitant or resistant to exploring consensual acts of domination and roughness in sex is completely normal. The prospect of controlling or being rough with someone, even consensually, can be scary. But there is a huge difference between dominating with coercion in a harmful way and playing a dominant role in a consensual erotic container.

As Midori puts it, "For the 'nice guys' and the 'nice gals,' the condition of engaging in dominance and submission may seem counter[-intuitive] to their internal morals or philosophy. I'm a nice [person]. I'm fair. I'm just. I listen. I collaborate." But, she adds, "This part of you can be incorporated in the conversations before play happens. Discussing boundaries, safe words, what kind of mood you're wanting to explore—by having a little collaboration at the beginning, you can acknowledge your inner good guy or good gal with the intention of playing the villain for a temporary period of time."

For those with "nice person" syndrome, it can be helpful to remember that the act of taking the time to get really clear on the wants, needs, and boundaries of anyone involved before the sex happens *is* part of being a considerate partner. You or your partner can remain (as the questioner put it) a "lover" during the process of negotiation, and if the two of you agree on some form of alternative play, you can take off that "nice person coat" during sex and put it right back on immediately after. This is why sex is referred to as "play"! It's an opportunity to have fun while surveying new sexy activities with your partner. The roles you take on when erotically engaging with others do not have to be permanent representations of who you are in everyday life.

In the context of BDSM, approaching sexual negotiation in a playful way by inviting your or your partner's affectionate "lover" self to join the conversation or scene is a great angle to initiate action. You can implement tactics to lean into your desires in an authentic way, even if one of you is interested in a particular style of play and the other is not. If you're looking to be dominated but your partner is hesitant, perhaps they could start off playing the hot stranger who makes a direct pass at you, while you take on the role of a submissive college student saying something like, "I know you want me but you're going to have to work for it." Or maybe your partner takes on the role of the dominant professor who shows you they are in control. The choices of scenes are endless; it's just a matter of working together in a well-informed, intentional way.

The more you and your partner(s) combine your visions, the better job you'll be able to do at harboring alignment and safety during play. Midori gives an excellent example of what this might look like: "Let's say you want to try bondage and you tell me you like being tied up. I would then ask you something like, 'When you're ready to be tied up, what will I see and hear? When it's not feeling good for you, what do you look or sound like?' And as the person performing the bondage, I would also share what they would see and hear when it's feeling good or uncomfortable for me. It's important to show each other what you look or sound like when some form of play is not feeling good for you. If you choose to use a safe word, tell your partner you still want to know what they look or sound like before you even get to the point where they must use their word. This doesn't mean you don't want them to voice their safe word, but it's helpful if they can show you what you could see and hear because it offers a more efficient way to salvage the experience if necessary."

It's important to take the time to actually talk this out, even if you are not exactly sure what this scene would be like. Midori recommends making your best educated guess. She says, "If your partner desires rough sex, and you ask, 'When you're envisioning rough sex, what will you look or sound like?' if your partner answers with 'You'll know it when you see it,' my response to that is *no*. Please don't resort to shirking responsibility. It's okay for someone to say, 'I'm not sure, but my best guess is my eyes will be squinted shut because I tend to shut my eyes when things start to feel uncomfortable. Or maybe I'll be chattering as a way of managing the discomfort. I could be wrong, but that's my best guess.' And then explore from there." The complicated nature of this process underscores just how crucial negotiation is to having a successful and fun sexual experience.

And not only is negotiation respectful and beneficial, but it can also be arousing. It serves as an invitation for you and your partner(s) to share more ideas about the sex you want to have.

Consent 2.0 aka Enthusiastic Consent

In negotiations like these, considering consent is vital. However, Midori suggests going beyond just consent, by first setting "enthusiastic consent" and then "collaborative consent" as the ultimate goal: "There's consent, and then there's enthusiastic consent. The next level is engaged, collaborative consent. In other words, are we equal partners in this? Or is this a one-sided negotiation where I asked for your enthusiasm and now you feel like you must give it back to me without sharing your own desires? Collaborative means discussing: 'How are we going to do this?' Who's Batman? Who's Catwoman? Who's doing the topping? And so on."

Pre-play talk creates more clarity on how you intend to play with your partner in a safe, enjoyable environment. When Batman enthusiastically agrees to top with a sharp understanding of when Catwoman needs to stop or slow down, Batman can relax and drop into the experience. The same applies to Catwoman, who can trust in Batman's ability to look out for their well-being. To put it simply, the more fearless sharing of needs, the better.

However, there is no guarantee that the conversation will go smoothly—in fact, it may even feel awkward or silly, especially while you're still developing the skills to communicate within this new, unfamiliar, and edgy topic. Midori advocates embracing the awkwardness because scenes in sexual play don't always go as planned. As she puts it, "With engaged, collaborative consent, all parties are now responsible for showing up on the playground together, and these conversations can be silly, fun, and sexy. The conversation could go something like, 'What if I were the pizza delivery guy and showed up at your door with a baseball cap, a hoodie, and a pizza? Ding-dong. *Did you order a pizza?*' You open the box and instead of a pizza, out comes a dildo with a harness. It's silly yet exciting. There's an opportunity to feel aroused and excited because it's so unexpected, and you can also laugh at the craziness of it all. But that's play! If you end up acting [a certain role-playing scene] out and you lose track of the plot, resulting in messy sex on the floor, that's still a win. Even if Batman doesn't wear his cape or the goodies in the pizza box weren't used, you still had fun." There's always next time to try this scene again or act out another one.

As Midori suggests, it's helpful to maintain an open mind to what's unraveling in each moment. Even if you or your partner(s) agree after negotiating to try something new, challenging feelings may still arise. This is when safe words and body language as a means of saying "stop" or "press pause" become important. It's imperative to always stay present throughout the experience, advocate for your needs before, during, and after play, and continue to check in with your partner(s), especially when it comes to engaging in new, adventurous, and potentially risky ways of play.

Give Expectations the Middle Finger

It's important to keep in mind that even with ethical, consensual communication, there's no guarantee that you and your partner will always be on the same page when it comes to exploring and meeting each other's sexual desires. The clever tagline of the Bonobo Network, a sex-positive learning community in California's Bay Area, sums this up perfectly: "High possibility, low expectation." This doesn't mean you're putting your needs on the back burner. Instead, it's about being honest with yourself and what you're hoping you might receive. If your expectations are very specific, you could end up disappointed with the end result even if your experience was positive. Keeping your mind open can lead to more positive outcomes for everyone involved.

 To learn more about negotiation, safety, and consent in highly sexually charged environments, listen to episode #256, "Sex Parties Aren't Just About Sex—with William & Misha of the Bonobo Network."

BE A SEXUAL SELF-ADVOCATE

As we've stressed so many times before, communication is key to healthy relationships with yourself and others. Asking for what you want is a huge deal that can be especially difficult when sex and desire are involved because it necessitates a mutually appreciated level of vulnerability. But vulnerability isn't something that happens automatically. It requires a conscious effort and the ability to get uncomfortable. If you find yourself struggling to ask for what you want sexually, challenge the belief that you're not supposed to talk about it. Sexual self-advocacy is one of the most important steps you can take toward having the fulfilling pleasure you deserve. Now is the time to confidently speak up and forge ahead to become the communication champion that you are. Go on—you've got this!

Are We Broken?

The stark truth is, most people in relationships—especially the long-term ones—will ask a variation of this question at some point in their lives. *Are we too different? Is this the right person for me? Is there any-thing we can do to salvage our relationship? How can we fix what feels broken?* Even if the sex and intimacy in your relationship seem healthy most of the time, there may still be moments when this question pops up. This chapter is meant to provide you with options on all points of the relationship spectrum. Whether you're figuring out desire discrepancies, mitigating relationship tension, considering consensual nonmonogamy, or looking to break up in a healthier way, this chapter can be the light at the end of the tunnel (or your life preserver on a sinking ship).

DESIRES AND NEEDS IN (LONG-TERM) RELATIONSHIPS

In Chapter 3, we discussed how lasting intimate connection requires a combination of newness and independence. It's common for people to find themselves wanting more. More novelty, variety, depth, connection, and varying forms of intimacy. Sex during the first part of a relationship is usually steamy and plentiful because there's freshness, excitement, and lust for each other. But what once was hot and exciting can become familiar and mundane. As a relationship goes on, it's expected for couples to experience a drop in sexual frequency and passion because the habituation of domestic life removes the obstacle, which decreases desire. And remember, just because you're married or living together doesn't mean things will be easy or that your partner is yours and yours only—even if you signed papers and exchanged vows, you still can't own a person or control how they feel or act.

As Esther Perel's work explores, the definition of desire varies from person to person. For many, desire is primarily about sex. For these people, questions like, *Am I wanted and desirable sexually?* or, *Does my partner find me sexually attractive?* may be especially important. For others, desire is geared more toward intimacy, making questions like, *Does my partner even value me?* or, *Do they care about my wants, feelings, and needs?* more significant for achieving fulfillment in the relationship.

DIFFERENCES IN CORE VALUES

It goes without saying that each person in a relationship brings their own unique combination of core values and life experiences to the table. Your sexual core values (the aspects of your being that seem like an intrinsic part of who you are) could be things like waiting to have sex until marriage, having a relationship style such as swinging or polyamory, being intentional about having sex frequently with your partner, or only having sex when true connection is felt, and so on.

So how do core values differ from wants and desires? Wants and desires can also be core values but are often lighter and more fluid, while for most people, their core values can feel like they're set in stone. Do you want to explore anal sex but are okay if it's off the table as long as you feel fulfilled in the other ways you engage in intimacy? Then anal sex is (most likely) not a core value. But, if anal sex is something that feels essential to you in your erotic landscape, then it probably is a core value. Differentiating between your inherent core values and your acquired wants and needs is up to you, but part of being in partnership is knowing these can differ from your partner's.

You can absolutely find yourself in a relationship where core values do not match even after "preliminary research" has taken place (such as dating and taking the time to get to know each other). You may also discover what once felt aligned now feels like a complete mismatch after a few weeks, months, or years. This does not necessarily mean you're doomed and have to leave the relationship. Instead, it's an opportunity allowing you to take inventory of yourself and the partnership that you chose to enter in the first place.

 Turbo-charge your confidence in speaking about sex with your partner in episode #265, "How to Talk to Your Partner About S E X—with Dr. Nan Wise."

I WANT MORE SEX (VARIETY, FREQUENCY, CONNECTION) THAN MY PARTNER

I love my partner, and we've been together for many years and have two children. However, our sex life is barely thriving. My partner is religious, and most things outside of traditional penetration are off the table. I've tried talking about having more variety, but it never goes well. I really don't enjoy sex because I can feel the lack of interest from my partner, but I don't want to force something they don't want to do. I've thought about infidelity and told my partner about it, but it didn't seem to matter. Are we totally broken or just incompatible? I cannot do anything to hurt my family. Please help!

According to Dr. Nan Wise, religious values or shame from a religious upbringing can be a common source of difference in core values. However, she says, in this situation, "people can be educated. They can get curious. There are books they can read, podcasts to listen to, and other tools out there to understand more about their sexual differences. [Building] passion in a relationship comes from taking some risks. It's not about the sex positions you use; it's about your willingness to go to challenging places with your partner and yourself—where you are relating to each other instead of living in that dead-end relationship." Thankfully, there are options to try for mismatched desires like this, so chin up and don't lose hope just yet, especially if you think your relationship is worth the effort.

It's About What You Do with Your Desires

In Chapters 3 and 4, we laid out how to understand and voice your wants and desires, and how to advocate for them with honesty and enthusiastic consent. As stated before, even if you know what you want and how to express it with clarity, you can still encounter hurdles with differing needs. But it's important to make an effort. As Dr. Nan puts it, "You never know what might come up. Your partner's perspective may be very different from your own. This may be how they perceive you as a supportive partner, or that airing everything out opens the door for more." However, when you do your best to share your needs in a loving and proactive way and are still met with a hard no, it may be time to make a pivotal (and possibly difficult) choice on how to further proceed with the partnership.

Let's approach the proverbial elephant in the room and talk about infidelity. Some people call it disloyalty, cheating, duplicity, or an affair, and however you choose to label it is entirely up to you, but the fact is, it can happen in relationships, and it hurts (usually for everyone involved). Both Amy and April know firsthand the pain and lasting damage that can come when truth has gone out the window in a partnership—especially when cheating is coupled with lying, gaslighting, inauthenticity, and questioning someone's truth. We both experienced nonconsensual nonmonogamy, and though we do not condone nor condemn people who share (or have shared) intimacy with others outside of their relational agreement, we advocate for integrity and honesty. This is because it can take an unfathomable amount of time to repair the damage that infidelity causes to a partnership, and sometimes it may be totally irreparable.

171

I WANT MORE SEX (VARIETY, FREQUENCY, CONNECTION) THAN MY PARTNER

1. Are you struggling with a partner who is uninterested in exploring your desires, no matter how much you've emphasized how important your needs are to you? If so, continue to read this chapter.

2. Do you want to find ways you can talk to your partner about your desires and needs, or aspects of your inner self, to understand other alternatives beyond what you've applied before? If so, continue to read this chapter. Also, go to page **148** of **Chapter 4: How Can I Ask for What I Want or Even Talk About Sex?** for the CONNECT formula, which can help you engage in these difficult conversations.

3. Do you want to learn ways to create a safer environment where your partner can uncover their erotic needs too? If so, go to page **219** of **Chapter 6: How Can I Become a Better Lover?** to add more tools to your erotic tool kit. (Remember: these tools are about showing up for your partner in a bigger and better way, *not* a manipulative means to getting what you want. Check in with yourself to be sure you're walking this path for the right reasons.)

One Person Cannot Meet All of Your Needs

For much of history, marriage had a pragmatic social function. It ensured economic stability and social cohesion and was based not on choice but rather on rules and obligation. People modeled their relationships by what they saw from their parents or members of their community. But in modern times, that paradigm has shifted. Now, most individuals (hopefully) have the ability to negotiate with their partner about what matters in life—like where you want to live, if you want to have children, or even when to have children. The choices are endless.

Esther Perel's work emphasizes that (spoiler alert!) *you truly cannot have everything you need in your life from one person.* There is no one person who will always be able to fulfill your every need, be your best friend, passionate lover, trusted confidant(e), dependable, predictable, and still supply you with mystery, excitement, and adventure. It's virtually impossible considering the different minds, bodies, upbringings, histories, and so much more at play between every individual. While it's helpful to be in a relationship with someone where your core values are aligned, you cannot seek out or expect one person to fulfill your every need for the long haul.

It can be beneficial to ask yourself a few questions about your relationship nonnegotiables, such as: *What needs feel crucial to be met specifically within your current relationship container? What needs or desires can be met elsewhere?* Can the idea of having more variety in adventurous experiences expand beyond your partnership? Are you willing to try new activities, such as joining a book club focusing on erotic novels, checking out a clothing-optional spa or retreat, or going out dancing to engage with others in a connective and even intimate way? Once again, the decision is entirely up to you. Within the container of consensual monogamy, each of these questions also optimally involves a larger conversation with your partner.

Negotiation 2.0

We've already started equipping you with some tools for better sexual communication in Chapter 4, but it never hurts to have more in your tool kit. In a situation where a partner is considering infidelity, Dr. Nan emphasizes the importance of speaking with honesty and attentively listening to your partner's feelings and needs. As a first step, she suggests trying to be open in communicating with each other. "This requires one person to take the risk and tell their partner how they feel, and it's their job as the partner holding these feelings to let the other person know how important pleasure is for them, and how essential exploring something [new] is as well." She also shares how desiring a passionate connection or seeking new sexual experiences within a partnership is not at all uncommon.

Since it's on each person to take the risk by telling their partner how they're feeling, consider also involving professionals, such as a sex or couple's coach or therapist. A skilled professional can create a safe environment to discuss differences and fears and help these conversations become as productive as possible. By doing this, Dr. Nan says, "Instead of having a breakdown of the relationship, you may be able to create a breakthrough and a better understanding of each other." (We'll delve into how to seek professional support later in this chapter.)

What If Your Partner Is Still a No?

You can say with as much clarity and intention as you possibly can, "Honey, I love you, and I really want more sex. I want to explore more variety with you," and if this is met with avoidance, defensiveness, or a cold, hard no, you could decide to throw in the towel and tell yourself just how hopeless it all is. But what if your partner did not pick up on what you were trying to convey, or they weren't able to accept just how important this is to you? Perhaps they think it's trivial, a phase you're going through, or simply something you will "get over" in time. Retrospectively, this may be how they *want* to see things, because this vulnerable conversation can bring up a lot of their own personal judgments and insecurities about you, themselves, and your relationship.

If you value your relationship, there are a lot of possible steps to take to mitigate your relational differences, including expressing how important your pleasure is to you, opening up about your inner erotic landscape, discussing how you've fantasized about others during sex, or taking a bold leap and telling your partner how you've contemplated being with other people because you haven't felt like your needs are being met even when you've lovingly discussed them. These conversations *will likely* be hard—even in the most passionate partnerships. But remember: If you want a change, it's imperative to put it all on the table.

Here's a short recap on the CONNECT formula from Chapter 4 to help you with these potentially terrifying conversations:

CONNECT:

1. **Consideration.** Approach when things are positive.
2. **Outside.** Have the discussion outside of the bedroom.
3. **Negotiation.** Ask for permission to talk about it.
4. **Nicely to the nitty-gritty.** Start with the positives and be authentic.
5. **Exposure.** Be willing to be vulnerable and expose your truth.
6. **Curiosity.** Elaborate on your curiosity and focus on the *we*.
7. **Therapy.** Seek a therapist or coach.

At this point, you may be thinking (although we hope not), *What if my partner is still a hard no after I've tried everything?* It could be that they are resistant to trying new things, unwilling to talk about sex or the relationship, or simply reluctant to seek outside support. Then what do you do? If you truly believe you've done *everything* possible to convey the importance of your feelings while offering your partner the opportunity to work with you, then this could be the turning point in terms of considering all potential solutions, and it might be the time to ask yourself some crucial questions. Do you stay and suppress this part of yourself while knowing that it does not just disappear and it could manifest in other ways, including further disconnection, dissatisfaction, and even resentment? Do you think that the differences in your relationship are too much for you to stay any longer and it's time to make the decision to leave? Do you propose a solution beyond the others and try again with some form of nonmonogamy? Or do you get your needs met outside of the relationship without the consent of your partner, realizing the same deepened disconnection, dissatisfaction, and resentment will likely continue with this choice?

Cheating, Affairs, and Nonconsensual Nonmonogamy

In late 2021, April was watching a movie and cuddling with her long-term partner when suddenly her friend barged into her house and confessed to having a six-month-long intimate affair with April's partner. Needless to say, that confession was debilitating to her. The ripple effect of the deception and dishonesty of her partner's act impacted not only April but also her friends, family, coworkers, and anyone who knew her. April was also immensely embarrassed and ashamed. With all the communication tools available to her and her partner, why would this still happen?

Relationships can be a total clusterfuck. But they can also be transcending and worth the hard work. April knows firsthand because she chose to move forward with that partner to try and start again. While she knew there were no guarantees for what to expect in the future, she trusted that they could find a way to rebuild their relationship.

Regrettably, this situation is not uncommon. The research of sexuality and relationship scientist Dr. Zhana Vrangalova, as well as other academics, shines light on the varying motivations behind seeking sex and intimacy outside of a relationship. Biology is only one part of the equation. People choose between monogamous and nonmonogamous relationship styles because of factors like the need for sexual novelty or greater frequency of sex, adventurousness, unalignment of desires, attraction to other people, and more. These things are very normal. In fact, Dr. Zhana theorizes that more than 90 percent of people in monogamous relationships will experience desire or attraction for someone other than their partner at some point in their lives.

When you add feelings of being unheard, unappreciated, unimportant, or misunderstood to those factors, it can cause turbulence in any relationship. This is where some people begin to consider cheating and nonconsensual monogamy as an attractive option—particularly when one partner is unable to meet the needs of the other(s) in a consensual way.

 Normalize your curiosity around nonmonogamy in episode #238, "Nonmonogamy and How to 'Open Smarter'—with Dr. Zhana Vrangalova."

In the face of a "relationship storm," we strongly recommend taking other paths before straying outside your relationship agreement and breaching the trust that was built. Why? Because infidelity can result in magnified shame and deep hurt for all parties involved in and around the relationship. However, if you choose stepping outside of your relationship in a nonconsensual way, consider a harm-reduction approach. For example, it is much riskier to your partner and your social community to have secretive sex with a neighbor or someone within your friend circle than to hire a sex worker, flirt on the internet or social media, or have virtual sex with a webcam model. (Modern sex tech even offers toys that allow you to have virtual sex with cam performers and porn stars.) If you do have in-person sexual encounters outside of the boundaries of your relationship, protect your partner's physical safety and health by using protection and being vigilant about the risk of transmitting STIs. It's the very least you could do for your partner, especially if you're continuing to have unprotected sex with them.

Nonmonogamy 101

Dr. Zhana has dedicated much of her career to researching nonmonogamous relationship styles. Specifically, her research suggests that purist monogamy—the traditional relationship, where people enter it thinking, "I will only want to be with this person for the rest of my life"—is actually far from the desired norm. A 2020 poll from YouGov asking people what their ideal relationship style is on a scale from completely monogamous to nonmonogamous suggests that around 50 percent of men and 35 percent of women would prefer some level of nonmonogamy or are unsure what type of relationship dynamic they prefer. Yes, you read that correctly, a significant percentage of people are *not* completely set on monogamy as their preferred relationship style. Although it's difficult to say how those same individuals would feel about their *partners* having occasional intimate experiences with others, these statistics show that desiring something outside of the traditional container of monogamy is completely normal.

Consensual nonmonogamy (CNM) is when a person engages in sexual activity with someone outside of their relationship with their partner's consent. CNM relationship styles vary greatly based on the individuals involved. They can include anything from having sex in the same room as others, to don't-ask-don't-tell situations like hall passes and "anything goes in different zip codes," to swinging and open relationships that are more about sex than connection, to non-labeled open relationships, to "relationship anarchy" where there are little to no rules, to polyamory where both sex and lasting connection are part of the equation . . . the list of CNM styles goes on and on.

The Stigma Around Consensual Nonmonogamy

The majority of cultural representations of family life and romance generally involve monogamous partnerships, and CNM relationships are often depicted as messy or unstable. This stigma has caused those partaking in CNM to keep quiet in fear of being judged or ridiculed. But here's the thing: most of the negative sentiment is based on outdated, prejudiced, and simply inaccurate assumptions about CNM—not to mention an unconscious bias towards monogamy as the gold standard for relationships (especially in the US). But recently, more people have been taking a closer look at nonconventional forms of romance and sex. Recent research has revealed that many individuals in various forms of CNM are doing very well—and even flourishing. With a growing awareness of these outdated stereotypes, society will hopefully continue to become more accepting toward the diversity of relationship styles.

Dr. Tammy Nelson, author of *The New Monogamy* and *Open Monogamy*, points out that both monogamy AND nonmonogamy can mean different things for different people. Is watching porn or having cybersex or webcam sex breaking your monogamy agreement, or is it considered safe and within the confines of your relational boundaries? If it is included, does that make you monogamous or nonmonogamous? And what about flirting, hugging, cuddling, kissing, holding hands, massaging, or even masturbating with or around other people? Everyone has their own definition of what being monogamous means to them. Hence, it's crucial to have conversations about it with your partner(s). You can outline what kind of relationship dynamic you want and talk about boundaries and how to define them. Determine what to do if there is a shift in boundaries and consider the best way to make these difficult conversations ongoing, open, and easy.

Both Dr. Nelson and Dr. Zhana also believe that certain forms of nonmonogamy (including cheating) are not always related to differing desires or disconnection. In truth, many people just love or need newness. Some of these individuals may want it with one partner, while others want it with more than one partner. Similarly, some want nonmonogamy to fulfill certain needs that are not available with their partner—for example, when one person is really into BDSM while their life partner simply is not, or when partners have differing desires or ability levels. Also, for many folks, distance can be an issue, and when they're living in different locations, sharing intimacy outside of the relationship makes sense to them. Other people seek out nonmonogamy as an opportunity for both individual and relational expansion because they find experiences with different people to summon more vibrance, aliveness, and a deeper connection with parts of themselves they had never experienced before. The most important part of this equation is, whatever the reason or method, the choice to break from monogamy is openly discussed and mutually agreed upon as a satisfying course of action for all parties involved.

 Reinvent how you think about relationships in episode #276, "Open Monogamy: Recreating Your Relationship for Hotter Sex and Connection—with Dr. Tammy Nelson."

Breakups Suck

Let's talk about a topic that's far from pleasant: breakups. Amy and April have been through many breakups in all their years on the planet, and the hurt and grief never seem to get easier. The ending of a relationship takes a toll on your inner well-being—whether the breakup is amicable or a devastating mess.

If you are finding yourself in a place where breaking up seems like the only option, consider viewing it as a transition to a new way of being, where valuable opportunities are on the horizon. Though this will likely be a difficult period, it is also a time to build a deeper understanding of yourself, cultivate more aligned relationships with future partners, and even enhance connections with friends, family, and/or children.

> Find more ease as you navigate the treacherous waters of breakups in episodes #296, "How to Navigate Breakups and Heartbreak—with Dr. Alison Ash," #129, "Conscious Uncoupling—with Katherine Woodward Thomas," and #218, "How to Find Peace in Betrayal, Breakups, and Divorce—with Tammy Letherer."

I WANT MY PARTNER TO ENJOY PLEASURING MY GENITALS

I used to have a lot of shame around my genitals, but I've recently become sexually awakened. Unfortunately, my partner feels differently. He is not into giving oral sex or focusing on my pussy in general. When we discussed this, the response did not feel good. It was along the lines of, "I just don't like doing that." I've expressed my desire for mouth and finger stimulation before sex, and, although it seems at the time like I'm being heard, nothing changes. Why doesn't my love want to pleasure me? He certainly enjoys penetrative sex. Is this a deal breaker, or is there something I can do?

Regrettably, this is an era where much of the world continues to glorify the cock while shaming the pussy. Even the clinical terms for the pussy can be unpleasant to the ear: vagina, vulva, clitoris, labia. Add to those some downright defaming slang and nonclinical terms such as ax wound, pink taco, snatch, gash, twat, beaver, cooter, clam, cunt, FUPA, or beef curtains (seriously, WTF!?), and you can begin to understand this disappointing reality. Some people, like April, were raised with parents who called it the "no-no," meaning this area is a no-touch zone . . . which can often lead to masturbation shame.

Shameless Sex prefers to use "pussy" to reference the vulva. If this word is off-putting to you (like "ax wound" is to us), feel free to insert whatever terms you like for your genitals. If it's the word "snatch" that strikes your fancy, and you feel on top of the world when you say, "I can't wait to feel your mouth on my snatch," then more power to you and your snatch!

Like many vulva owners, neither Amy or April was educated on how to refer to our bits. However, to us, at this point in time, "pussy" feels right. Now both of us say "pussy, pussy, pussy" all over the place, including restaurants and airport bars (where we have to remind each other to lower our voices to avoid offending anyone that still prefers to call it their "no-no"). For Amy and April, "pussy" is an all-encompassing word, whose meaning extends from the inner and outer labia to the almighty clitoris and its extensive parts, to the vaginal canal and leading up all the way to the cervix. "Pussy" is connected to pleasure, empowerment, orgasms, aliveness, sensation, and beyond. For further encouragement on loving and owning how you view your genitals, check out Bodysex, a practice designed by the late sexual pioneer Betty Dodson, where Carlin Ross (the "keeper of all things Betty Dodson") and other certified Bodysex leaders teach Dodson's methods of sexual pleasure and empowerment across the world.

Perfect Pussies, Penises, and Porn

Let's revisit one of the most influential and accessible sexual forces on the planet: porn. Remember, it should only be consumed for entertainment purposes, not for education. Most porn is not an inclusive or realistic representation of sex and its expansiveness, so it generally does not teach you how to have pleasurable and safer sex—nor does it show the vast diversity of how bodies look, act, perform, and respond.

Much of modern porn is made to glorify the cock and please a cock-owning viewer. Porn presents an idealized version of genitals, encouraging people to believe that what they're viewing is what the "perfect" bits should look like. Pussies, for example, should be symmetrical and have an even flesh tone, with small, tucked-in labia all flawlessly shaven and waxed, and the "ideal" penis should be somewhat girthy, at least seven inches long, neatly circumcised, and always hard. But news flash—this image is complete and utter bullshit! It is a well-supported fact that genitalia are as varying as fingerprints and snowflakes. This image of the "perfect" pussy or penis doesn't exist (for one, *nothing* on the human body is perfectly symmetrical). And if you're a human who likes to rock a pubic hair bush, then *do it!* Your pubic hair is there for a reason, including emitting pheromones and even preventing transmission of bacteria and other pathogens during sex. So power to the pubes—go ahead and let your hair down!

While porn is likely the primary culprit for many people's shame around the size, look, and performance of their bits, shame can come from many different directions. How your parents talked or (more commonly) didn't talk about genitals, what your peers said when you were naked in the locker room, or a sexual partner's critical comment about your bits all affect how you feel about your body. It's up to you to do the work to reframe the shame with compassion, love, and acceptance for yourself. Just remember that your penis, pussy, or anything in between is fucking fantastic, just like you.

 Reprogram your brain beyond what porn taught you about perfect genitals in episode #212, "Penis Shame: Size, Look, and Performance—with Soleiman Bolour."

I WANT MY PARTNER TO ENJOY PLEASURING MY GENITALS

1. Would you like to know your options if your partner is a hard no to celebrating your genitals? If so, continue reading this chapter.

2. Are you looking for more effective ways to talk to your partner about how their approach toward your genitals and your pleasure feels to you, or would you like to better understand their barriers? If so, continue reading this chapter. We also think revisiting the CONNECT formula on page **148** of **Chapter 4: How Can I Ask for What I Want or Even Talk About Sex?** could help you get more confident when having difficult conversations around sex.

3. Is your partner open to learning more about your genitals and how to touch and approach your bits? If so, go to page **208 of Chapter 6: How Can I Become a Better Lover?** for ways to pleasure all types of bits and for more items you can add to your sexual menu.

Both Amy and April have plenty of experience with lovers who were resistant to exploring their genitals outside of penetration. We've had partners who were closed off to pleasuring our pussies with their mouths as well as people who were highly opposed to anything anal. Sometimes these scenarios were major deal-breakers. Other times we found ways to meet these partners somewhere in the middle. The truth is, there are some people who will just be a hard no to various forms of pleasuring pussies, cocks, or assholes. This may be something that can change over time, or it may be an intrinsic part of them based on orientation, biology, past experiences with sexual trauma, or other scenarios.

Understanding Your Partner at a Deeper Level

Every person has their own set of unique preferences and core design built into them from birth. Unsurprisingly, there are certain things you can't change about an individual's identity. There is no way to "pray the gay away" (thankfully!). Equally, there's no button to press to delete someone's deeply rooted feelings or beliefs. In fact, any pressure to change the primary way your partner experiences consensual intimacy, as well as the hard nos on their sexual menu, will likely cause more harm and internalized shame.

Some aspects of sexual needs and desires are more preferential, meaning there is a possibility they can change—but only if the person truly wants to work toward these shifts and is ready to embark on altering their belief system. Let's use an example that has nothing to do with sex. Let's say a person just hates cold weather. They can't deal with ice, snow, frigid air, and freezing temperatures, so they avoid traveling anywhere with colder climates, assuming they'll be miserable and it'll be a waste of a trip. But then, one day, this person falls madly in love with someone who lives in the last place they ever wanted to be: Alaska. Despite their reluctance, this relationship becomes so important that this person does some research and they begin seeing Alaska in another way. While it's cold almost the entire year, it's a stunning place with incredible landscapes, loads of wildlife, and exciting new adventures to experience. The cold-hater decides to give Alaska a try, at least for a few weeks to see how it goes.

We can't say if that cold-hater chose to stay in Alaska to be with their lover in the end. But we do know that, regardless of the final outcome, making an effort, obtaining knowledge, and trying a taste of something you typically don't prefer can lead you to new places, unexpected experiences, and shifts in those old perspectives (in the bedroom and beyond).

Determining whether your partner's no is embedded in them or if it's a potentially workable matter of preference can be difficult. While it's still 100 percent up to them to decide if they want to shift and lean into your desires, there may be an opportunity to engage in open and curious dialogue to learn more. Have you had a deeper investigation into exactly what your partner is not interested in (for example, what your partner finds unattractive about your genitals)? Get specific with the inquiries: *Is it the look, the smell, the taste? How long have these feelings been present? Is it something they've felt for most of their life? If so, what was their upbringing like regarding sex? Did they ever have a challenging or hurtful experience with this type of sexual contact? What were the early messages they received about it? Is there anything you two can do together to create a space of open exploration where your partner is willing to try something new?*

Many people in the "deal-breaker" position only see two options: A) enduring an unfulfilled and unhappy relationship, or B) calling it quits and leaving the relationship. But have you ever stopped to consider options C, D, and E by digging deeper? Let's get curious and look at the other options that aren't so limiting.

DIYing Your Own Sexual Fulfillment

Option C might involve continuing to do your own work to expand your pleasure. Along the way, you can create opportunities to share your breakthroughs and knowledge with your partner, maybe even inspiring them to jump onboard. But beware: If you choose this path, you *must* be clear about your intentions and expectations. As psychologist and psychotherapist Dr. Nicola Amadora says, "You can only work with what is true right now." While you may hope your partner witnesses your continued sexual evolution and hops on your ship toward pleasure island, it may not happen the way you want it to. While hope can be a great source of fortitude and enthusiasm when attempting to make shifts, be careful about keeping your hope from growing into an expectation. Hope can transform any unclear expectations into unrealistic ones, resulting in distress and dissatisfaction.

If you decide to embark on this path, be honest with yourself and as transparent as possible about any expectations you have for your partner's growth. For example, you can make a commitment to doing two to three months of self-work and combine that with patience for your partner, whatever their pace is. Better yet, you can let your partner know how important this is to you by saying something like: "This is really big for me, and I'm going to continue to do my work, and my hope is that you will join me or at least attempt to do your own self-work. Can we be patient with each other and have a check-in about this in ____ days to see how we're both feeling about this?" If after that time, you're still not seeing any progress and the issue remains important to you, then it may be time to reconsider the relationship structure.

Remember, you can only work with what is true in this exact moment. Let that be a guiding force as you continue down your path, and never stop celebrating your fantastic, amazing, beautiful, unique, and glorious sexual self.

 Perfect the art of speaking to your truth in episode #101, "How to Have Deep Connection and Juicy Sex!—with Dr. Nicola Amadora."

Don't Be Afraid to Bring in Outside Support

Options D and E might involve adding professional support, which can be essential in some situations. Have you ever heard the saying "You can't teach an old dog new tricks"? Some people are "old dogs" with real limitations to learning and changing. Others are living in survival mode, where their system is too overloaded to deal with something new.

However, many people find that receiving guidance from someone other than their partner helps improve tricky relationship situations. What if you suggest looking for a therapist or coach who specializes in sex and relationships to help unpack your differences? As part of initiating the conversation to seek support, try using the CONNECT formula on page 149 to make it a "we" thing and not a "you" thing. If your partner agrees, then you can start the process of finding the right professional whom you both feel heard and safe with. If your partner responds with avoidance or resistance, perhaps because there is a common belief that therapy is "what broken people do" or "we're a strong couple who can figure this out on our own," then ask (or even insist) that your partner try at least one session and go from there.

If you and your partner are open to something outside of talk therapy, there is also a more experimental route you can take. You can find skilled professionals trained in various somatic therapeutic methods such as Somatica, Hakomi, and IFS, to name a few, who can guide you to better understand and appreciate each other's pleasure through safe and consensual exploration of one another's bodies.

 Deepen your knowledge about how to seek outside support with episode #268, "How to Find the Right (Sex and Relationship) Therapist or Coach—with Keeley Rankin, MA."

ORGASMS TAKE ME A LONG TIME, SO I FAKE IT

My partner and I are having a hard time in the bedroom. We're only a couple years into the relationship, and our sex life isn't doing so hot. It takes me a long time to orgasm. Sometimes I feel like it's too long, so I fake it. I don't understand why it takes me so long to cum. I've never used sex toys before and wasn't sure if I ever should because I don't want to become dependent on them. Is it me or is something wrong with us?

First and foremost, it's not your job to orgasm for your partner. Sex should never be a job unless you're choosing to do sex work (and if that's your jam, then make that money, honey!). The unforgiving truth is that a lot of people get stuck in a cycle where certain aspects of sex end up feeling like a job or a chore—especially in long-term relationships. Consider blowjobs. For starters, the name suggests it's a job, so that's a bit of a mindfuck all on its own. Secondly, while there are plenty of people who love sucking cock, it's not for everyone. For those who feel like it's a chore or something they "should" or "must" do, they end up offering it at obligatory times like birthdays, Valentine's Day, or as weekly, monthly, or even annual maintenance, where they aren't enjoying the experience, often waiting for it to be over the minute it starts.

This is just one of the many ways people engage in unenjoyable sex to keep their partner(s) happy. But what if it didn't have to be this way? For most people, the primary purpose of sex is to experience connection and pleasure, so what if you could *learn* to love sucking that cock, eating that pussy, having penetrative sex, and on and on?

Well guess what? *You can!* It will likely take some work with yourself and your partnership container, but there are paths to make these shifts. One huge step will be letting go of the idea that it's your job to perform a certain way just to please your partner. Whether it's faking orgasms or giving obligatory oral, don't "should" yourself into doing anything you don't really want to do.

Why Do People Fake Orgasms?

Both Amy and April have faked orgasms, and so have many our vulva-owning friends—as well as a few penis-owning folks who were willing to be radically honest about it. At times, faking orgasms can feel easier, especially when orgasm isn't happening and it feels like the clock is ticking. Eventually, we both learned how to advocate for our unique needs in the bedroom and realized what our bodies could experience when those needs around sexual pleasure were expressed and then met, ending the cycle of faking orgasms.

When we look back to why we chose to fake orgasms, it becomes clear that it originated in a general lack of knowledge about sex, an inability to speak about what our bodies needed for pleasure, and a fear driven by the desire to people please. It took us both a long time to get where we are now but, after dedicating a lot of work to developing full ownership of our bodies and sexuality, neither of us have needed to (nor have we wanted to) fake orgasms for anyone—ever again. This shameless truth can be yours too.

You hopefully already know it's not helpful to put your own pleasure on the back burner just to make others aroused. Instead of speaking up to ask for something that might feel more pleasurable, or requesting for the sexual experience to end altogether, many people are inclined to fake orgasms "to get it over with." It's important to note that it's definitely okay to do this if the situation feels unsafe or if you're still working on voicing your needs. Even though there's a different approach that can ultimately benefit everyone involved, it requires a lot of effort to overcome the habits, conditioning, and even survival mechanisms that keep you from taking this approach. So, if this is you, don't be too hard on yourself.

For vulva owners, especially those having sex with penis owners, part of the problem may be skewed arousal expectations. As we've discussed in Chapter 1, most vulvas take longer to receive the blood flow necessary for arousal than most penises. It's understandable why a complex internal organ such as the vaginal canal would take longer to get blood flow than an external body part like the penis. Think about the physics! The former has simply more volume to fill. Add to this fact that every person's bits are going to react in their own way, and expectations of arousal levels can often be downright wrong. Because of these differences, people start to believe that their desires are mismatched and feel pressured to match the expectations set by their partner's body.

Different people also are aroused by different things to begin with, both for individual and psychological reasons. For example, as Dr. Nagoski's work highlights, most vulva owners get a clit boner (yes, science shows clits get boners too!) in *response* to something rather than in anticipation, whereas most penis owners tend to experience arousal *before* desire—though this is a generalization, so it does not apply to everyone. When your arousal patterns don't seem to be matching your partner's (or what you think your partner wants from you), faking orgasm can *seem* like an easy way out of the problem in order to resist the potential repercussions of hurting your partner's feelings. But that avoidance technique can come at great cost to your future pleasure.

The Consequences of Faking It

When you fake orgasms to keep your partner happy, everyone loses. Not only do you lose your actual potential orgasm and the pleasure you deserve as a human being, your partner's understanding of your unique pleasure is also affected. It may seem like faking an orgasm is helping by boosting your partner's ego in that moment, but in reality, it's denying them the opportunity to learn more about your sexual fulfillment. Not to mention, if this relationship ends and your partner enters a new sexual relationship, they will probably repeat the same techniques thinking, *My last partner could orgasm from this [position, rhythm, etc.], so why isn't it working now? What's wrong here? Are we just incompatible? I don't get it*, and the problem perpetuates.

ORGASMS TAKE ME A LONG TIME, SO I FAKE IT

1. Do you want to figure out more about what your body likes and how to guide your partner in doing those things? If so, continue reading this chapter.

2. Do you want to learn how to talk to your partner about what you need and the pressure you feel to perform in the bedroom? If so, continue reading this chapter. We also recommend revisiting the

CONNECT formula on page **148** of **Chapter 4: How Can I Ask for What I Want or Even Talk About Sex?** so you can better handle these difficult conversations.

3. If you finish reading this chapter and you continue to have questions about your arousal and ways to explore your sexual pleasure on your own, then go to page **40** of **Chapter 1: Am I Normal?** so you can tap into your body and your orgasm.

4. Would you like to know more about how sex toys can enhance orgasm during partner play? If so, go to page **116** of **Chapter 3: How Do I Know What I Want in the Bedroom?**

The good news is that this may not be a compatibility issue. The two of you could be destined for a long, beautiful relationship full of great sex and lots of orgasms. But there is also some not-so-good news: You have some work to do to step into your sexual power. Let this book be your invitation because *now* is the time to take a stand and commit to your *Shameless Sex* journey. With this intention, it will be helpful to clue your partner in on what's been going on with your orgasms— including the fake out. Even if this sounds terrifying, it's a vital step in the right direction.

Sharing Is Caring (And Sometimes Terrifying)

It isn't a must, but full, honest disclosure can deepen your connection and improve the sex you're having. The road may be rocky, especially when you first open this conversation. Your partner might feel hurt, deceived, unworthy, or ashamed, and these feelings are valid. They may go through a process of believing something is wrong with them or that they're not a good lover, but that is not yours to take on. The first step, where you take accountability for your inauthentic orgasms, is yours, so remind your partner that you're initiating this dialogue for change because you love them and want things to be authentic. You may discover some repair is needed, especially if your partner feels like they've been lied to. If this happens and you find yourself unsure of how to navigate these heavy repair conversations, revisit the CONNECT formula on page 149. Also, if your partner starts to go down the dark rabbit hole of unworthiness, instead of coddling them, remind them that this is an opportunity for the two of you to discover more about each other. It's not a one-sided issue—meaning it's not just about them or you. And keep in mind: Once you get through the sticky, hard, emotional stuff, the wildly playful and fun exploration begins!

Batin' University

When you're learning (or relearning) how to find your O with a partner, we cannot emphasize masturbation enough. (There's a reason why we keep coming back to it!) Going on a masturbation journey can be extremely beneficial and even therapeutic. It's like going to college, but for a degree in pleasure and self-discovery. You'll learn to better understand what parts of your genitals like to be touched, how they like to be touched, and what gets the blood flowing to your bits. If your bits need to be rejuvenated, just flip back to page 41 in Chapter 1, page 86 in Chapter 2, and page 111 in Chapter 3 to get that batin' education. It's the key to unlocking much more than a few orgasms.

Incorporating sex toys into your private time is another way to potentially unlock greater pleasure. Sex toys are among the best ways to enhance yummy sensations within yourself and your partner(s), which makes putting a few in your sexy tool box well worth it. If you're new to sex toys, explore them on your own before adding any to partner play. That way you can get a feel for what types of toys you like, as well as the level of pressure, intensity, and places on your body you prefer to use them. For an introduction to the wild world of sex toys, including the myths around sex toy addiction, venture on back to Chapter 3.

The Genital Elevator

Batin' and sex toys are by no means the only ways to tap into your personal pleasure. But before laying out those other possibilities, let's revisit something stated a few times already: It is normal to need warm-up, foreplay, and connection before having sex. This is especially central for those with receiving orifices, but it's important for people with any bits or sexual roles. Think of sex as an elevator and foreplay as the button you press to enter that elevator. Removing foreplay is like not pressing the button and expecting the elevator doors to open. You can press the button and patiently wait for the elevator to reach your floor, but aggressively trying to pry the doors open (even when there's a slight crack) doesn't mean you can slip on in. That elevator must reach you before you can go anywhere.

So as scary as it is, remind yourself that building up to your pleasure, no matter how long it takes, is important. We encourage you to do your best to advocate for your own arousal within your capacity.

Shameless Sex's *Prompts to Pump Up Your Partnered Pleasure*

Hopefully by now you're at a point where you've opened up about your ultimate desires, creating the understanding for what you need to enjoy sex and intimate touch with your partner. Once you've got that foundation, the world is your oyster! Below are some tips for taking the next step to gratify your pleasure.

1. **Advocate for it**. Ask for more touch, kissing, connection, cuddling, and warm-up before anything goes near your genitals. Be assertive! If your partner makes moves before your body is ready, let them know you need more of Y before moving to Z. The simple formula from page 147 of Chapter 4 ("appreciation + AND + what you want") can go a long way. For example: *I love when you touch my clit AND I love it even more when we make out for a few minutes and then you touch my clit because it gets me even hotter.*

2. **Reframe it.** Part of shamelessly sharing your needs may also include expressing the pressure you feel to orgasm or perform a certain way. Consider asking your partner to join you in reframing sex to be about pleasure and connection, where orgasm is a bonus but *not* the final destination. There is no guarantee they will join you in the viewpoint, but at least they'll be aware of the pressure you feel and how it affects your sexual body (and your potential orgasms).

3. **Show it.** Regardless of how long it takes you to have an orgasm, if you're aware of what your body needs to get off, show your partner. Invite them to put a hand exactly where you want it. Then consider putting your hand on top of theirs and move it with the pressure

and at the pace you desire. You can also guide your partner in other ways. As sex educator and repeat podcast guest Samia Burton says, "Get your nut"—meaning, move your body against your partner's in a way that hits all the right spots. Everyone's way of "getting their nut" will be different. But your genitals may enjoy, say, more grinding as opposed to thrusting as a means of receiving increased sensation around your clitoris. As long as your partner is on board, take time to explore the positions that help you "get your nut." Don't be afraid to take the reins!

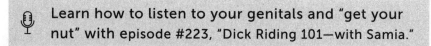

> Learn how to listen to your genitals and "get your nut" with episode #223, "Dick Riding 101—with Samia."

4. **Make it mutual**. Ask your partner if they're open to a mutual masturbation session. You and your partner may be able to see firsthand what each of you likes by masturbating while watching each other. Make an agreement about what the person who reaches orgasm first will do to support the other as they continue to do their thing. It could be watching, holding, kissing, rubbing, or whatever feels good. Just remove expectations, pressure to orgasm, and time from the equation and make it about mutual pleasure.

5. **Add it.** Start incorporating your hands and the sex toys you've chosen into your sexy playtime. If you know what drives you to arousal, start adding those things as well. Incorporate your hands on your body to see what feels good for you—maybe rubbing your clitoris, or massaging your testicles, or putting a finger in your ass. Whether you're penetrating or being penetrated or neither, this is about *you*

touching you while consenting to having sex with someone else, so wherever your hands go on your own body is completely up to you.

If sex toys are new to your bedroom play, have a conversation with your partner *before* sex. It can be as simple as: "I bought a sex toy. I'm super excited about it, and I think it would be fun to use it together." If you're concerned about your partner feeling inadequate or if you receive some pushback when you bring it up, use the "shit sandwich" technique: Put the hard shit you want to bring up in the middle of two complimentary things. For example: "I love having your cock inside of me, AND (not but) what I would love even more is if we could add this sex toy into the mix too. *It feels so good.*" If the response is, "No, why do we need that?" and it remains something important for your sexual well-being, then check out the other CYOPP options in this chapter on page 174 to learn what to do if your partner is still a no.

6. **Lube it (literally).** Often, the problem with unpleasurable penetrative sex is simply not enough lube. While lubing up does not guarantee you a ticket to O Town, nor should it serve as a Band-Aid for not feeling aroused, it most certainly can help things feel more enjoyable. Are you using enough lube during sex?

    If not, be sure to get yourself some high-quality lube. It's a must-have staple for anything from manual sex to sex toys to cocks to anal. No matter what you're doing, your body and your bits generally prefer *not* being met with a bunch of friction. As we've expressed before, *Shameless Sex*'s top pick is überlube because it's long-lasting, super silky, and feels amazing on your body. It never gets tacky and is less likely to throw off the vaginal pH than other lubes. It's just quality stuff. In our opinion, it's as good as it gets. If you're looking for a lube that's not silicone-based, check out Sutil or Sliquid's Organics Oceanic line.

7. **Lube it (metaphorically).** In the words of podcast legend and one of *Shameless Sex*'s biggest inspirations Dr. Emily Morse, *communication is lubrication*. When it comes to relationship challenges both in and outside of the bedroom, communication is key in rebuilding and repairing connection. There are no guarantees it will fix everything, and sometimes the misalignment can be so vast that repair is not possible. However, the very least you can do is *try* to have those deeper conversations to see what is possible. When you do, think of it as lubing up the dialogue so things can go a lot smoother and sexier.

SINK, SWIM, OR SAIL—YOU DECIDE

No relationship is perfect, and there are many reasons why you could become (or already are) less sexually interested in your partner—no matter how awesome they are. But before making any rash decisions like leaving or cheating, try to reframe your feelings toward your partner and make mindful efforts to identify and address any triggers that might be negatively affecting your relationship dynamic. Consider using the power of your words and committing to open and ongoing conversations about the issues. This is where you'll be able to map out your expectations and identify any commonalities that allow for a thriving partnership—or differences that initiate seeking alternative options.

If it comes down to leaving the partnership because it's sinking faster than the *Titanic*, do your best to depart with respect, decency, and integrity. Give them a hand to get into a lifeboat—don't let them sink! After all, you chose to be in a partnership with them for a reason. And most importantly, keep in mind that a breakup isn't a "failure" or anyone's fault. Sometimes you have to take a few steps back to see how to move forward. Do you sink with the ship, swim in the debris hoping someone will save you, or do you hop into the USS *Shameless Sex* lifeboat and sail into the next chapter?

6

How Can I Become a Better Lover?

I n this chapter, we'll concentrate on how to achieve sexual mastery by further tuning into yourself and your partner. Among the various topics covered on the *Shameless Sex* podcast, sexual mastery stands out as one of the most sought after. The high number of downloads for episodes like #107, "How to Eat Pu$$y Like a Champ," and #258, "How to Give Handjobs & Blowjobs That Will Blow Their Minds," is proof that most people want to become better lovers.

First things first: What is sexual mastery? It's the capacity of a person to connect with, and experience, their own body and desires in a way that leads to authentic and empowered self-pleasure as well as sexual connection with others. It's a process of exploration, discovery, and growth—a skill that you work on every day, and something that you can achieve. When you have sexual mastery, you'll feel more confident, brave, and self-assured so you can have more connected sex.

To quote George Leonard, author of *Mastery: The Keys to Success and Long-Term Fulfillment,* "Mastery is not a state to achieve, but a journey to live by." As he discusses, the consumption-driven and marketing-heavy society we live in is highly focused on persuading people to abandon mastery in favor of quick fixes. That's why *Shameless Sex* isn't offering you some magic pill to swallow or a three-step plan for becoming a sexual master. It can be complicated, and we can only guide you toward discovering what's right for you. There's no one right way to do sex and relationships, so the more you know about yourself and the possibilities available to you, the better your chances are of having enjoyable sexual experiences.

Even though this chapter primarily focuses on pussies and penises, the same principles can be applied to anyone with bits other than those as well. Now it's time to get your sexy on and start honing your skills so you can elevate your pleasure game.

I WANT TO PLEASURE THE PUSSY

I am in a relationship with a wonderful woman, and while I don't recall ever having issues pleasuring lovers in the past, my usual techniques aren't giving her orgasms. She's told me a little about what she likes, but whenever I try, nothing happens. I really want to give her the pleasure she craves. What can I do to make her orgasm and be the lover she desires?

Both Amy and April are no strangers to the pressure surrounding orgasm. For a long time, April equated her worthiness in the bedroom with her partner's orgasm. She would only consider it "great sex" when her partner climaxed—even when she didn't. If her partner didn't orgasm (because

204

she couldn't "make" them cum), she saw it as a failure and left the experience wondering what *she* could have done better.

Society sends a clear message: Any type of sex should lead to orgasm. And although applying pressure can be orgasmic on G-spots, prostates, and other erogenous zones, this performance pressure is *not* beneficial for giving or receiving pleasure. While we will be offering lots of tips for becoming a better lover, the focus will not be about *making* your partner(s) orgasm. Pleasure is subjective and individual, so you can't consensually *make* anyone do or feel anything—especially orgasm. The best you can do is encourage them to enjoy the ride and all the pleasureable sensations that come along with it—even if they don't reach the "finish line." After all, the journey can be just as satisfying as the destination. In fact, many people relish the journey of sex, loving all the delicious feelings and sensations that happen from beginning to end, orgasm or no orgasm. Think about a pleasure scale that goes from one to ten. If you ride that scale somewhere between a six and a nine (between enjoyable, really fun, and fucking hot), you're still going to have a great time even if you never hit a ten (the Holy Grail of orgasm). This is what enjoying the journey looks like. And in fact, once the pressure to get to the Holy Grail is taken off the table, givers and receivers often find sex to be connected and gratifying anyway because their minds are more fixed on what is happening in the moment.

If Pressure Were Poison, Presence Would Be the Antidote

Pressure can be a real buzzkill when it comes to sexual performance and orgasm, but there's a remedy: presence. We've said it before and we'll say it again—being present with your partner, conscious of the moment, and aware of yourself by being connected to your body and the person you're engaging with is one of the key elements of sexual pleasure *and* mastery. Think of pressure like poison in sexual experiences and presence as its antidote.

Presence is something both Amy and April continue to work on nearly every day. Without training, your complex brain rarely chooses to slow down and step outside the internal mental vortex. When you're in your head thinking about your insecurities, remembering tasks you need to complete, feeling numbness or struggling with sensation, you are disconnected from presence. If this is you, this is not your fault in the least—there are a lot of reasons why presence might be difficult for you. But all these presence barriers are workable. With enough practice, you'll be able to one day finally flip the presence switch. It can be deeply rewarding in many ways—and will even make you a more attuned, badass lover.

The Orgasm Gap—and How to Close It

As mentioned back in Chapter 2 (page 92), the "orgasm gap" has been around for a very long time. A study of sexual behavior published by *The Journal of Sex Research* in 2014 (and repeatedly reinforced by current case studies) indicates that less than 30 percent of vulva owners reach orgasm during PIV sexual activity, whereas over 90 percent of penis owners usually do. Since clitoral stimulation is the most reliable method of reaching orgasm for the majority of vulva owners, PIV sex that doesn't engage the clitoris often doesn't result in orgasm. Moreover, various studies of sexual behavior and beliefs revealed that vulva owners in relationships with penis owners tend to prioritize PIV penetration and the penis owner's satisfaction even if it means sacrificing their own pleasure.

One of the first steps toward creating more equitable pleasure is deceptively simple: communicating and listening. In general, communication in which one partner is able to articulate their sexual needs to another who's receptive to their needs is instrumental to a more satisfying sexual relationship. In *Psychology Today*, Laurie Mintz, PhD, discusses a few more essential ingredients to mutually fulfilling sex. First, vulva owners (and their partners) must understand that the clitoris is key to reaching orgasm—even in PIV sex. Second, people engaging in PIV sex have to treat clitoral stimulation and penile stimulation as equally important.

I WANT TO PLEASURE THE PUSSY

1. Do you want to uncover the art of sexual mastery when it comes to pussies, expanding on ways you can become a better lover to go above and beyond in meeting your vulva-owning partner's sexual needs? If so, continue to read this chapter.

2. Do you find it challenging to let go of the idea that it's your responsibility to bring your partner to orgasm or that it defines your self-worth? Is this belief causing a roadblock in your life that you're struggling to overcome but wanting to move through? If so, continue to read this chapter.

3. Do you feel like you could use more understanding as to what your partner wants during intimacy? Have they given you some clues, yet you still want to know more but aren't sure how to approach the topic? If so, go to page **148** in **Chapter 4: How Can I Ask for What I Want or Even Talk About Sex?** and use the CONNECT formula to tackle tricky conversations around sex.

So you want to be the master of pussy pleasure, and it's clear you're choosing this path for yourself just as much as for your relationship? Fucking fantastic! Go grab your rain jacket and galoshes because it's time to get soaked in all things pussy pleasure.

Mastery Through Sex Hacking (Starring the Dual Control Model)

Former Kinsey Institute director Dr. John Bancroft and Dr. Erick Janssen developed a concept called the Dual Control Model of Sexual Response (this is relevant to pussy pleasure, trust us—your patience will pay off). This model focuses on the differences between sexual inhibition and sexual excitation, as well as how they interact with one another in creating both mental and physiological turn-ons. As Dr. Nagoski puts it, this model offers a simple but radical shift in the way you think about turning your partner on, involving not only adding stimulation but also slowing down or stopping to generate more safety and relaxation.

Kenneth Play, vulva pleasure expert and author of *Beyond Satisfied: A Sex Hacker's Guide to Endless Orgasms, Mind-Blowing Connection, and Lasting Confidence,* sums up the "dual controls" of the Dual Control

Model: "One system is telling you about what you shouldn't do and inhibits you, while the other one excites you." In order to have a sexually fulfilling experience, Play suggests "lower[ing] anxiety to lower inhibition—but the situation also has to have a level of excitement." This can be a tricky balance. He continues, "Every person is different in what arouses them in an erotic context. Some people love a partner who's very patient and soft in the beginning, but when you get down to sex, they want more animalistic or dominant energy." In the moment, this might seem confusing, but the Dual Control Model actually provides an explanation. In Play's words, "It's important to understand that there are two phases of [your partner's] experience. Phase one is about creating safety, and phase two is about creating excitement. The key that I've found, from my own research and sex hacking, is to drive up as much arousal as possible [in the safety phase] so you aren't trying to start from scratch."

The Dual Control Model is just one aspect of brain function that Kenneth Play's work explores. As an innovative sexual educator, Play teaches tools called "sex hacks" that help you become a better lover by learning about and applying the way the brain works to deliberately discover and refine your sexual skills.

Despite humans' shared brain structure, Play stresses that each person's needs vary. For example, every person is different in the amount of accelerator and brakes they need in tapping into their ultimate pleasure—and part of sex hacking, and achieving sexual mastery, is taking these differences into account and even exploring them to find out what brings your partner(s) the greatest potential for pleasure.

With vulva owners, this can be especially difficult. As Play explains, "Sometimes you are doing everything right physically, but you're not doing it with the energy [your partner] wants. If you don't understand [their] erotic mind, then you're not bringing the right energy that would be arousing for [them]." To successfully please a vulva owner, it can be crucial to learn to move with the ebb and flow of your partner's ever-shifting wants and needs. As Play puts it, "You can learn how to surf those waves. So, when it comes to those orgasmic positive sensations, like the ocean, you can't force it."

As professor of neuroscience and psychology James G. Pfaus, PhD, says, "The erotic body map a [vulva owner] possesses is not etched in stone, but rather is an ongoing process of experience, discovery, and construction which depends on [their] brain's ability to create optimality between the habits of what [they expect] and an openness to new experiences." Or, in other words—sexual pleasure is complicated! It can take a lot of learning to figure out what makes a person tick sexually.

Paying Attention to the Pussy

To become the ultimate pleasure giver, it is crucial to pay attention to your partner's body and needs. Look for the subtle shifts the body naturally makes when it likes or dislikes something. For example, when Amy's partner is pleasuring her pussy with his hands or mouth, she'll mimic how her body feels with her hands. When she's relaxed, her hand lies flat on her chest or grazes her body with desire. When things start to feel more intense, tickly, or "too much," her hands start to clench up. Her knuckles make a fist to brace for the feeling she is experiencing. This is just one example, though, and each body is different. Some people show their arousal (or lack thereof) through their toes, eyes, hips, even redness on their skin, while others may not give any visible signs at all.

For this reason, take moments with your partner to check in. If you see their hands clenching or if you feel a shift in your partner's sexual energy that confuses you, use this as an opportunity to touch base with them. Approach with curiosity and openness. You can say something like, "I love having my mouth all over your pussy . . . I'm also noticing your hands clenching. Just curious if that means anything or if you'd like me to do something differently." If you're the receiver, respond with your truth. For example: "If you see my hands clenching, that means I'm on the edge between comfortable and uncomfortable. I'll do my best to voice this when it's happening, but if you see me do this, please check in with me." This type of communication is easier said than done. However, every time you can voice your needs in the moment or share what you know to be true about your body before sex happens, you will likely have more connected and pleasurable sex than if you hadn't.

Sometimes, it can be even better to have this conversation outside of the bedroom, when people are not naked and feeling vulnerable. You can even schedule weekly or monthly sex-life check-ins. Set aside a time when you're both feeling grounded and available to talk about sex. Begin with the good stuff and follow with what you're wanting more or less of. You could say something like, "I'm really loving that we're having these sex-life check-ins, and I'm learning so much more about what your body likes. AND, one thing I'd love is more verbal foreplay, where you tell me how much you want me and how sexy I am. Also, one thing I'd like less of is your mouth on my bits before your hands have spent some time warming me up. Oh, and can we try incorporating more lube into our sexy time too?"

Apart from being attentive toward your partner's needs, it's important for you to know how to be mindful of the sensations you are feeling. The more you focus on a particular area of your body, the more you can feel. If you don't believe it, just close your eyes and try tapping into a specific part of your body. Your left big toe, your right pinky finger, your upper lip. Don't touch or move that part, just simply notice the sensation happening. Now imagine doing this with your hands, mouth, cock, pussy, and all the in-betweens.

This is especially important for people with receiving barriers or sensitive genitals that have been grabbed, poked, or prodded in the past. It can be easy to get accustomed to things happening too fast and with more intensity than your body is ready for—even when it diminishes your pleasure. So, as you're exchanging touch with your partner, remember the *Shameless Sex* mantra: *Go slower than slow, then slower than that.* You and your partner may not even be aware of just how much slowness can enhance your pleasure.

Sex educator Midori recommends something she calls "the pussy hug." Bring your hand to the pussy, and before you do *anything,* cup it, hold it, hug it, letting the pussy and the human who owns it know you're there to take your time and consider their pace. This also allows the skin-on-skin touch and differing body temperatures to acclimate to each other. Once this has happened, then you can move your hands ever so slowly to other areas.

We know that slowness can be hard to practice. April, for one, has got a bit of a lead foot, even in the bedroom. To counteract this, she considers her sensual adventures like a stroll instead of a race. Taking your time can really pay off; you can soak up all the smells, sights, and sounds if you just slow down. Even if you're the type who craves instant gratification like April, slowing down in the bedroom can help you to appreciate all the special details unfolding between your sheets.

The Top Three Erotic Must-Haves

As you explore pussy pleasure (or any pleasure), there are three main things you should keep in mind to take your sexual experience to the next level.

The first erotic must-have is to **remove goals.** Don't go into things with a specific goal in mind. Not only will goal-seeking put pressure on you and your partner(s), but it may also distract you from your partner's actual needs and desires. Kenneth Play makes a great point when he says that you should always have your partner's best interests in mind and prioritize their well-being over anything else. By throwing goals out the window and focusing on your partner's needs instead, you will be able to "create a safe container for more arousal to happen."

Continued foreplay—the second erotic must-have—is just as crucial, if not more. Part of prioritizing your partner's *well-being* also means putting it before your own desires (and we hope your partner would do the same for you). Play likes to look at foreplay as more than just the activities you do *before* penetration—it's about generating excitement and potentially giving your partner multiple warm-up orgasms beforehand. This helps them relax and be more aroused, which can lead to more pleasurable penetrative sex. As he puts it, "We should be less concerned about premature ejaculation and be more concerned with premature penetration!" This holds true for people not engaging in PIV sex as well—whatever you and your partner(s) desire, make sure that everyone's minds and bodies are ready for it.

It's important to remember that the body holds limitless possibilities for erotic stimulation. There's no need to concentrate on just one part of the genitals or even just on the genitals at all. As French sexologist and author Gérard Leleu so eloquently put it, you can give your lover the best possible experience by "playing the whole keyboard of orgasms." The orgasmic opportunities are limitless, so why play only a short and simple song when you can create a full-blown symphony? Play agrees: "As long as you keep switching up the songs, [your partner] will keep responding. But once you find something that works, don't fuck with it. Continue with what you're doing until it's over or they want to do something else."

But what happens after you play the whole keyboard of orgasms with your partner(s)? Do you just put the instrument aside and call it a day? Or can you take in all the feel-good endorphins of the experience you just created together? Whether they scream and wail with pleasure or they hang out on a more moderate level, there is an opportunity to nourish and adore the dynamic beauty of what just occurred. Within the sexual world, this is called **aftercare**—the all-important third erotic must-have to keep in mind.

Play explains that aftercare is about showing your partner that you truly care for them. To ensure they have a positive experience, help them transition back to earth after flying to the moon. This does not just stop at the physical act; it's about creating a space for them to relax and enjoy their pleasure. Play even recommends saying, "You don't need to manage anything. I got this." He believes this is one of the most satisfying things you can express in the moment so the other person doesn't slip right back into management mode.

Aftercare is a gift to anyone you have the opportunity to be intimate with. For many people, sex and sensual connection are deeply vulnerable experiences. So why not celebrate it . . . not once, but every time you engage in intimate experiences? Even if your partner does not have multiple mind-blowing orgasms this time around, the aftercare you provide can remind them they are safe, loved, and appreciated no matter what happened. Who knows—it could even create more opportunity for deeper connection and hotter sex the next time around.

 Go "beyond sex" and master pussy pleasure in episode #272, "A Sex Hacker's Guide to Endless Orgasms and Lasting Confidence—with Kenneth Play."

Shameless Sex's *Go-Tos on Giving and Receiving*

After you've got the basics down of removing goals, extended foreplay, and aftercare, you can take your intimate encounters to the next level. It's time to learn about intentional giving and receiving: one of the most game-changing practices for becoming a better lover. This technique will not only help you sharpen your giving skills, but it will also let you know more about your partner's body. Many of the steps below are similar to what we discussed in Chapter 3, in *Shameless Sex's Ways to Stimulate Self Pleasure* on page 111—only this time, the pleasure is for someone else.

- **Schedule intimate time.** Try exploring giving and receiving nights (or whatever time of day fits into your schedules) with your partner. Life is busy and there are lots of interruptions, like children, work, and social media. But try picking at least *one day, every week* and set aside thirty minutes (or more) to explore uninterrupted intimacy with each other. Each time, determine who will be the sole receiver and who will be the sole giver and then swap periodically, so the giver does not receive in the same session as they give. You can switch roles whenever you decide to, but staying in one role for a decent amount of time will provide you with more benefits than switching often.

- **Share requests.** If you need more direction as the giver, ask your partner to make two requests for what they'd like to receive before entering the sensual space. Remember that requests are not demands but instead an open opportunity for negotiation. If your partner says, "I definitely want a lot of kissing on my lips and all over my body, and I'd also love to play around with some spanking on my ass," it's up to you to decide if you're able to meet those requests. And respond accordingly: "I am a big yes to kissing you on your lips and all over your body, and right now I'm not in the spanking place, so is there a third or fourth request we can add to tonight's menu?"

  Another possibility is to make an agreement to take penetrative sex or any genital touch off the table completely. If the receiver gets to a place where they're saying, "I need you inside of me NOW," take a moment to check in with them to understand if their system is having a hard time receiving or if they actually need some gentle encouragement to relax and let go. Maybe they do need to get railed at that very moment because they are so in their arousal. Whatever the case, you choose how to navigate this, but understand that as the giver, you are taking on a powerful role of holding space for whatever arises for the receiver. It may be orgasms and passion, but it could also be an emotional roller coaster of pleasure mixed with tears, anger, and frustration. Be prepared to hold it all while maintaining your own boundaries.

- **Embrace receiving barriers.** If you're the giver, let your partner know that this time is all about them, and they don't need to do anything except receive, communicate, and guide you as the giver. Let them know that you're just happy to be there focusing on their pleasure. As you are giving, you might encounter "receiving barriers" from your partner. These often come up when either a partner feels uncomfortable or unfamiliar with the touch they're experiencing, or they have conditioning around worthiness where they feel like they need to "do something." When this happens, just press pause. Stop what you're doing and invite them to check in with themselves to find out what they really want at that exact moment. Approach this pause with kindness, compassion, and patience. Their answers could vary from "I have no idea" to "I just want to be held" to "I want your hands on this other part of my body with light pressure." Drop back in and try to meet them in whatever capacity they need (if it's within your own boundaries, of course).

- **Pamper your partner.** Perhaps you draw your partner a hot bath and massage their feet and shoulders while occasionally looking into their eyes and telling them how much you care about them. Maybe you wear an apron and cook them a delicious meal, wash the dishes and then invite them to relax as you sensually massage their entire body. This can lead to erotic touch, and even genital touch, but it doesn't have to. The trick is to get creative and think about what would feel good for *your partner*. This probably will differ greatly from what would feel good for *you* as the giver, but it's not about your pleasure during this round.

- **Save the genitals for last.** If you do make it to the genitals, explore genital massage first rather than going right for the bits where people often get stuck on orgasm as the goal. Genital massage is less about orgasm than it is about providing pleasure and sensation. If you've ever had a massage from a trained massage therapist, try to mimic that experience. They will slowly warm up your body by first taking their well-oiled hands and gently placing them on your body without moving. Then when they start to move, they go slowly, using their entire hands from the palm all the way to the tips of the fingers. When they make their way to your shoulders, they rub and knead and work the tissue in a way that should feel enjoyable and deeply relaxing. The same techniques can be applied to the bits.

  When you first begin to incorporate this practice, keep your fingers out of any orifices unless the receiver asks you to enter them. In fact, even beyond the context of genital massage, anytime you're entering an orifice such as a vulva or anus, take your time to warm up the external body before entering them. When you think the moment is right to take things further, be sure to ask your partner if they are ready for penetration. If you get the green light, put some lubricant on your finger (or cock or sex toy) and rest it lightly on the opening of the vagina or anus for a minute, then gently make your way in. Taking it slow is the best way to go. You may even be able to sense your partner's receiving orifice opening up and pulling you in, but only if they are totally comfortable.

Sex Toys and Sexual Mastery

If you and your partner are down to add sex toys into playtime, then know this is an easy way to enhance your sexual experience. If sex toys are difficult for you to wrap your head around, consider this an opportunity to reframe your mindset. Why is it important for the pleasure you provide someone else to come solely from your body? Where did you learn this, and what is the driving force behind this need? Pleasure is pleasure, and if your partner gets aroused and orgasms from sex toys, this should be something to celebrate! If you're ready for increased good vibes by moving past the idea that your mouth, fingers, and cock are the only things to get the job done, then go to page 116 in Chapter 3 to learn about the best vibrating sex toys to have in your erotic tool box.

 Let us help you find the right sex toys for you in episode #200, "Our Favorite Sex Toys."

Why Do You Need to "Make" Your Partner Orgasm?

Remember April's story about feeling like she needed sex to end in orgasm to be satisfying? Well, eventually with a bit of effort and awareness, she learned to revise her sexual agenda and replace those orgasm objectives with sexual self-exploration. Since then, all aspects of her sex life have improved (for real!)—from the intensity and frequency of her orgasms to the sensation and connectedness during sex, even when the sex hasn't resulted in orgasm. This is an example of what can happen when you remove goals from your sexual equation.

The first thing to do is check in with yourself about *why* it's so important for you to "make" your partner orgasm. When did this belief start and where did it originate from? What if your partner says they are perfectly happy hanging out at six or eight on the pleasure scale, and they would prefer to enjoy the journey with the Holy Grail of orgasm as a bonus? Can you get on board for enjoying the depths of pleasure and connection without needing to have an end goal? Thinking about these questions can help you be intentional in the way that you think about sex. Embracing sex when the goal is simply pleasure and discovery can unlock a world of erotic possibilities. Plus, you can't "make" anyone do anything. The decision to unlock their pleasure is entirely up to them.

I WANT TO CONQUER THE COCK

I'm married and want to be more confident, seductive, secure, adventurous, and shameless when it comes to sex with my penis-owning partner. We live a busy, stressful life, but I still want to become a sexual powerhouse and master that cock. How can I create sexy nights and spontaneous fun experiences to broaden our sex life?

Whether you've got one or you love one, becoming a sword master is possible. There's no magic to Excalibur, but there are some tools to help release that sword from the stone (and overcome daily stresses while you're at it).

If you don't own a penis, mastering cock pleasure can be confusing and even daunting at times. There will be some trial and error involved, and even when you believe you've become a master cock pleasurer, your partner's needs can still change over time. But masters don't give up. Author and educator George Leonard said it best: "There are no experts. There are only learners!"

Practice Builds Confidence

At around twenty-eight years old, when April was finally ready to give oral again after her first nonconsensual experience with a blowjob in high school, she lacked any sort of confidence or know-how. She was riddled with insecurity and doubt and would shyly avoid exploring anything that resembled her past trauma. In the end, she was able to build confidence by going to workshops, studying different techniques, and learning how to vulnerably communicate her oral experiences with her partners in real time. She told each partner she chose to "suck off" that she was there because she felt safe and secure with them and because it felt good for her to pleasure their cock. She also would state her boundaries by saying, "No pushing my head down, no deep throating, and I need to be in control," and then she would ask her partner to verbalize what did and did not feel good for them. This type of honesty opened an erotic floodgate that continues to evolve her cock mastery skillset to this day.

Ready to follow in April's footsteps and dip more than just the tip into the how-tos of cock mastery? Time to CYOPP to become the prince of the penis, the duchess of dick, and the countess of cock with proficiency in pleasuring that penis (aka the D).

I WANT TO CONQUER THE COCK

1. Do you want to gain tools to further tap into your own sexual badassery so you can show up with complete confidence in bringing your penis-owning partner into erotic bliss? Do you want to expand your knowledge of ways to deliver pleasure to the D? If so, continue to read this chapter.

2. Do you want to find out how to fully speak your true desires and let your partner know how much you want to become the conquerer of their cock? If so, continue reading this chapter. We also recommend going to page **148** in **Chapter 4: How Can I Ask for What I Want or Even Talk About Sex?** and using the CONNECT formula to guide you through asking for what you want during sex.

3. If you want to discover even more ways to spice up your sex life, go to **Chapter 7: How Can I Have a Hotter, Steamier, More Connected Sex Life?** for an array of options and ideas to turbo-charge your sexual menu. We also recommend you continue reading this chapter.

Cock Mastery Starts with You

When it comes to becoming the ultimate giver (no matter what bits you're rocking), your own journey is equally as valuable and important as your partner's. After all, you are the one pleasuring that D. This means considering your own needs, comfort, and boundaries as you take your lover to new heights of decadent sensations.

When it comes to handjobs, or what award-winning sex educator and coach Ashley Manta refers to as "hand sex," positioning is key to conquering the cock. Her favorite hand sex position is what she calls the "reclining diamond." It involves the penis owner lying on their back with their legs spread like a V while you sit in between their legs with your legs resting on top of theirs. If you have a hard time visualizing this position, just think about the shape of a diamond. This position's benefits include less fatigue, easy access to your partner's bits, and the possibility for both the giver and the receiver to have full use of their hands.

Ashley also emphasizes the importance of remaining comfortable throughout the experience. Prop yourself up with pillows or a backrest if you need it, and when discomfort occurs, switch positions. As the giver, your comfort is just as important as that of the receiver. When you are free of physical distress, you will be able to be more present, drop into the experience more fully, and be totally on your hand sex A game.

 Harness your skills as a hand sex master in episode #114, "Handjobs—with Ashley Manta."

Being comfortable applies to any type of sexual pleasure you're giving, including with your mouth. Changing positions or slowing down to tend to any neck and back pain, as well as accounting for distress in your jaw, is crucial when you're giving oral. If your jaw gets tired, press pause and take a break by using your hands or even some cock-tastic sex toys. If you have a small mouth or suffer from TMJ (temporomandibular joint disorder, which can cause pain with jaw movement) like April, focus your mouth on the tip of the cock while putting your well-lubed hands around the shaft at the same time. This provides the receiver with a similar experience to having your whole mouth wrapped around the cock but still tends to your body's needs and capabilities.

Both giving and receiving pleasure have one thing in common—YOU. Alicia and Erwan Davon, experienced sex and relationship coaches and repeat podcast guests, agree that the key to pleasuring someone else is for you to be turned on while authentically enjoying the experience. Be there because you truly want to be, moment to moment.

 Glorify your giving skills in episode #258, "How to Give Handjobs & Blowjobs That Will Blow Their Minds—with Alicia and Erwan Davon."

The Davons' Penis-Pleasuring Pointers

The Davons provide some terrific tips for delivering penis pleasure, whether you're using your hands or your mouth, that apply to givers of all bits. While these pointers concentrate on hands-to-cock techniques, you can also apply them to oral pleasure because just about anything you do with your hands can be replicated by your mouth in some way.

- **Be in your arousal first.** Before pleasuring someone else, connect with your own genitals so you're turned on as well. If challenges arise, focus on your body, your turn-on, and what the touch feels like while it's happening versus the result. If you're unable to get into your arousal, then it might not be the right time to pleasure that D. It's important to engage only when you are truly up for it, and stay in it for as long as it feels right.

- **Think about rhythm.** Create a nice smooth rhythm—not super fast, but not too slow—and take little half-second breaks, so the receiver doesn't ejaculate really quickly or numb out. Over time, gradually increase the pressure, then bring it down again, creating larger and smaller "peaks." A rapid change in rhythm during a handjob or a blowjob can be jarring and tends to bring the receiver's arousal down.

- **Use both your hands.** Stroke the shaft and the head, but don't forget about the testicles or the bottom part of the cock. Stroke the cock with one hand while the other hand is cupping the balls or stroking the bottom part of the cock that's hidden. The hands are doing two different things. Having variety between your hands, like using heavier pressure with one hand and lighter pressure with the other, creates a pleasurable counterpoint. The heavier pressure is relaxing and more grounding. The lighter pressure is stimulating and exciting.

- **Do sensuality research.** If you're at a loss as to what to do, explore. Give yourself the opportunity to discover what you like by doing what the Davons call "sensuality research." In other words, have some fun and figure out what you enjoy, rather than allowing your inner critic to take over and rush through it. After all, doing it right is simply having a great time with your partner.

Cock Conquering 2.0

If you really want to take your blowjob skills to the next level, sex educator and creator of the #MouthMasterclass Samia Burton has the playbook to help take your blowjob skills from blowjob 1.0 to blowjob 2.0 so you can go full throttle on that stick shift.

First, she recommends that you get to know the cock in question. If you're getting down with someone new, ask, "How do you want your cock sucked?" If they're a consistent partner, check in every now and then to see if they have any new direction. Try sucking their cock with a few strokes and then asking what they like in your most sultry, curious voice. If they don't have an answer, offer suggestions. "Do you want long tongue strokes? Short ones? More pressure? Less pressure? Faster? Slower?" As Samia says, you are the Dick Tailor, designing the ultimate experience for you and your partner. Since you're probably not psychic, get to know what that cock (and the human connected to it) likes by proactively communicating about it.

Once you've got a sense of what that D needs, go to work! Being aroused involves blood flow into the genitals, and the longer arousal continues, the more pleasure ensues. When your mouth is going up and down the cock, you're pulling the blood upward and then pushing it back down again. Think of the upward motion as expanding your partner's pleasure by pulling it outward, and the downward motion as allowing the enhanced blood flow you just created to remain in the cock. Whenever you're on an upward motion, try incorporating a tighter grip with your mouth and hands to increase stimulation, and when you go back downward, loosen up and use less pressure.

Next, it's time to think about edging—or continuing to build arousal while delaying orgasm. What are the signs they're about to orgasm? Does the cock get harder? Do you feel their cock pulsating right before? Do the balls tighten up closer to their body? Does their leg twitch, or is it something they say? Pay attention and do your research. That way, if they're getting close and you want to continue to build up their arousal, you can slow down and do something else, and then ramp it up again. The more layers you add to their turn-on, the stronger their orgasm may be.

All that's left is cheering your partner on to the finish line! Encourage them to breathe when they're about to orgasm. Not only will it help them stay in the moment, but it will also likely make their orgasm even stronger (because orgasm follows blood flow, and blood flow needs oxygen). Invite your partner to take long, deep breaths as they sail to O Town. If you're feeling really adventurous, cheerlead them on with your most sensually sexy voice.

 Take your oral game to a whole new level in episode #237, "Oral Sex 2.0: #MouthMasterClass—with Samia."

Cock Conquering 3.0

By now you have an abundance of options for how to conquer the cock with your mouth and hands, but what about when it comes to riding that dick? Here are three shameless ways to ramp up pleasure when it comes to PIV sex.

- **Be adventurous with the cock.** Play with variations of movement that feel comfortable yet pleasurable for you and your partner. Go beyond the typical in-and-out movement of thrusting or the back-and-forth motion of grinding. Instead, try any (or all) of these techniques: swirling your hips in a circular motion; taking your sweet time and going as slowly as possible to build their arousal while working up to faster and harder; riding that D to the beat of your favorite sexy songs; and painting an infinity sign with your pelvis. The key is to be creative while paying attention to the technique(s) that turn them on but in a way that also feels fantastic for your pussy.

- **Hypnotize the cock.** During any form of PIV sex, imagine your pussy swirling around the head and shaft as if it's a vortex trying to suck every inch of their cock inside of you. Do this by focusing your energy on your vaginal canal, envisioning it spiraling upward (toward your head) with every movement. Where attention goes, energy flows, and their cock, along with your pussy, will likely respond accordingly . . . just ask Amy because this is one of her favorite techniques.

- **Massage the cock . . . with your pussy.** Kegels (the contractions of your pelvic floor muscles) can serve as a hands-free massage tool for your lover's cock! Try tightening and releasing those muscles during penetration to heighten sensation for both you and your partner.

Happy Endings

Sexual mastery can help you craft your own happy endings in the bedroom. As long as you remember to be intentional, learn to play your partner like an instrument, and think outside of the box, that fairy-tale finale can be yours (and your partner's). Applying the sets of skills and practices laid out for you in this chapter will help you become more attuned to your body and sexual energy. But keep in mind that sexual mastery is not something that can be achieved in the blink of an eye. It's a practice—or more like an an ongoing adventure—and it always starts with you.

The better a lover you become, the easier it is to learn how to have hotter and more connected sex, which we'll delve into in the next chapter. But it's important to walk before you run, so be sure you feel well versed in the diverse language of sexual touch that's covered in previous chapters before moving forward into these juicier aspects of sex and intimacy. And, if you're ready to forge ahead into the land of passionate possibility, then turn the page. It's time to cook up some enticing new dishes for your sexual menu. Let's get your mouth watering and those sensual taste buds tantalized! We hope you're hungry for what's next.

7

How Can I Have a Hotter, Steamier, More Connected Sex Life?

After you've learned about sexual mastery, it's time to add more hotness, eroticism, passion, and connection in the bedroom. This can be especially relevant for people in long-term relationships, where partners *think* they know each other forward and backward, and their curiosity lessens. Many times, people find themselves wanting more—more newness, variety, depth, and varying forms of intimacy. What once was arousing and exciting can become familiar and mundane.

Chapter 5 highlighted *why* connections fade and relationships lose their spark, but now it's time to jump into how you can reignite the fire within yourself and your partnership(s). This chapter is all about play, celebration, exploration, discovery, and the sexy things that get your juices flowing. Whether it's by indulging in fantasies and role-play, experimenting with kink and BDSM, exploring threesomes, or being open to new techniques and activities in the bedroom, this chapter is designed to help you find the fuel to pour on that fire burning inside of you so you can keep things hot in your sex life.

TALKING ABOUT SEX IS HOT!

Talking about sex can be difficult (and for some, downright terrifying). However, with enough practice, it can also be utterly *sexy*. A lot of people are interested in mastering the art of dirty talk (aka sexy talk), so think about discussing your sexual desires as a form of dirty talk all on its own. This may include many different things—the ways you prefer to be touched, new sensual and sexual practices you'd like to try, even asking questions about your partner's desires. Not only can these conversations lead to hotter and more connected sex, but they can also act as a catalyst to heat things up in the moment. So, embrace the dirty talk and let the sparks fly.

Again, we recommend talking about trying new sexual activities *outside* of the bedroom and most of the sex experts we've had on *Shameless Sex* agree. Discussing desires at a nonsexual time and even on a different day than you actually get it on decreases the likelihood of challenges or triggers arising from the vulnerability of that conversation. So, keep your pants on, ask your partner if they are open to talking about sex, and take a risk—knowing some sexy magic will probably follow. If you're not sure where to start, go back to Chapter 4 and revisit the CONNECT formula as well as the other helpful tools for having conversations about sex and relationships.

Spice up your bedroom talk and strengthen those sexy conversation skills with episode #277, "How to Add More Hotness and Desire to Your Relationship—with Dr. Lori Beth Bisbey."

MOVE BEYOND GETTING THE OLD SPARK BACK

Before diving into the glorious world of how to have hotter, steamier, more connected sex, remember that sex and relationships are always fluid and ever changing. So, fueling a "spark" in your relationship is less about "getting that old spark back" and more about re-creating, redefining, and reigniting a *new* spark. As founders of the Somatica Institute Danielle Harel, PhD, and Celeste Hirschman, MA, say, this often involves adding new items to your sexual menu. As you become less attached to the way things once were and begin to explore the endless possibilities of what is available and achievable, you may discover something that feels even more arousing than anything you've experienced in the past. Grab some popcorn and a box of candy (or better yet, a ball gag and some lube) because it's time to let the sex games begin!

 Find out how to expand your sexual menu in episode #133, "How Core Desires Lead to Hot Sex—with Celeste and Danielle."

I WANT TO SPICE THINGS UP AND FIND NEW WAYS OF BEING SEXUAL WITH MY PARTNER

My partner and I have pretty good sex, but it's been getting more and more routine as time goes by, and I want to spice things up. I have a growing curiosity about butt play, Tantra, kink, role-play, threesomes—I want to try it all! We've discussed this before, and my partner seems aligned in most of my interests, but I want to proceed in a way that feels really good for both of us. What is the best way for us to move forward?

Your sexual menu is a list of all the things you want, don't want, and are open to trying during sexual exploration. Your menu will constantly change as you learn about your unique desires. Often, people structure their menus in some form of a yes, no, and maybe list.

Creating a sexual menu is a valuable asset in keeping the fire burning (and for just knowing yourself better). Not only does it provide more clarity to your internal desires and boundaries, it also helps your partner gain a deeper understanding of what knocks your socks and underwear off in the bedroom (and beyond). If all parties engaging in sexual intimacy know and share their sexual menus, you just might have the perfect recipe for some mind-blowing sexy time.

The process of creating your sexual menu is easy. All it takes is you, a pen and paper (or a cell phone, computer, or even a voice recorder) and some space to consider your sexual wants and needs. Then think about these questions: *What sexual practices resonate as something you need or definitely want to do? What are you open to but unsure of? What actions or behaviors does your gut instinct say "fuck no" to?* When it comes to spicing things up in the bedroom, your yes and maybe lists are a treasure chest in terms of finding new, creative ways to play, and your no list informs all parties of what might feel hurtful, triggering, or challenging for you at this point. With that said, it's important to align your yes and maybe lists with your partner's to ensure their needs are taken into account as well.

Feels Good to Be (Consensually) "Bad"

Let's face it, for many people, the taboo of what *not* to do can be super enticing, and "taboo" forms of play like kink, BDSM, and anal often show up on people's sexual menus. But with that said, taboos often require extra communication, presence, and boundary setting to make sure everyone is as safe as possible. We suggest educating yourself before trying out taboo or intense sexual experiences, especially if they are new to you, by focusing on resources from accredited professionals. As kink educator and expert Orpheus Black states, taboo practices like kink "[require] an abundance of education, trust, communication, and safety [as well as] in-depth discussions about needs, desires, and boundaries with play partner(s). It's not something to dive into without doing your research, [and] it's not something to be taken lightly, so the more knowledge and communication, the better."

What If Your Partner Is a No to Your Yes?

You may discover a few of your yeses are on your partner's hard no list. If those yeses are important to you, more discussions may need to happen. This is when you give coercion the middle finger and invite curiosity in.

You can ask your partner why these acts are a hard no for them. What about them sound uncomfortable, scary, or like they're just not their thing? Are there options to create and explore a variation of your yeses in a way that feels safe while honoring your partner's nos? For example, let's say you want to explore anal pleasure with your own ass, and your partner is a hard no to this. Do more investigation: Does this mean all anal pleasure is entirely off the table, or can fingers and/or anal-safe toys be integrated? And if that's also a hard no, what about you using your own fingers and toys on yourself during your playtime together? There are plenty of ways to work together to compromise with each other in some way, but everyone has to be on board during the negotiation process.

I WANT TO SPICE THINGS UP AND FIND NEW WAYS OF BEING SEXUAL WITH MY PARTNER

1. Do your combined lists of yeses and maybes in the "things to try" category of your sexual menus include anal play (anything from toys and fingers to pegging and prostate play)? Or do you want more insight into what types of anal play are out there to experiment with? If so, continue to read this chapter.

2. Do your combined lists of yeses and maybes in the "things to try" category of your sexual menus include kink, BDSM, role-play, or Tantra? If so, continue to read this chapter.

3. Are the shared yeses and maybes suggesting curiosity in playing with others including threesomes, group play, or other variations of nonmonogamy? If so, continue to read this chapter.

4. Would you like a refresher on how to navigate fantasies? If so, go to page **131** in **Chapter 3: How Do I Know What I Want in the Bedroom?**

Anal for All

Everybody has an ass. It's the universal orifice, also known as the booty, back door, sphincter, butthole, or bum. Even though it's often regarded as taboo for sexual contact, the anus is packed with nerve endings and has massive potential for pleasure. Hundreds of millions of people either enjoy or are curious about anal play (enter Amy and April raising our hands with defiant smiles because we both *love* some backdoor action).

However, you must remember: Anal is not for *everybooty* (sorry, we couldn't resist). There are people who do not wish to explore anal play, and that is a preference that they are entitled to. In addition, many people specifically choose to avoid it because they have had negative experiences with some form of anal stimulation. This might include a visit to the doctor for a rectal exam, a nonconsensual act of sexual violence, or even an unpleasant previous experience trying anal that was painful (maybe due to accidental slippage or not enough warm-up time, preparation, or lube). Add hemorrhoids, surgeries, prostate issues, ass gases, and the fact that most people are picking up anal how-tos from porn, and it's no surprise why a lot of folks have an aversion to anal play. If this is your partner's position, it's important to respect it.

If you're a person who does want to try anal, it's also important to remember that there's lots of variation between asses and between what each of those asses need to have pleasurable sex. It's a fact that the ass's

Anal Structure - Vulva Owner

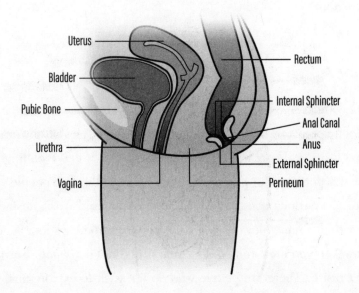

Uterus

Bladder

Pubic Bone

Urethra

Vagina

Rectum

Internal Sphincter

Anal Canal

Anus

External Sphincter

Perineum

anatomy is similar no matter what bits you're rocking. But just like breasts, penises, vulvas, and all parts of the human body, *everybooty* is different. From the shape and size to the look and feel, every ass is unique in what it wants and needs. However, penis owners have an extra asstastic treat within. The prostate—an erogenous zone that can be accessed through the anus—is especially pleasurable.

We'd like to clear up a common (but silly) misconception for any straight men out there: Anal play does not make you gay. The ways people like to play are not at all correlated with their sexual orientation. This means if a straight man enjoys pegging (when a vulva owner anally penetrates their partner, generally a penis owner, using a strap-on dildo), this does not mean anything about his orientation. Orientation is about the

Anal Structure - Penis Owner

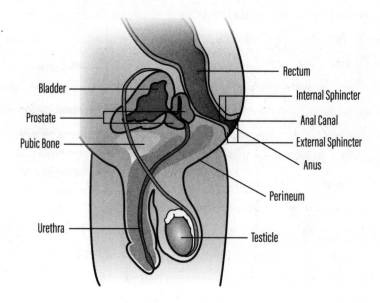

people or genders you are attracted to and interested in having sex with, not about the actions or behaviors you partake in.

Now that we've got that out of the way, it's time for the fun stuff! If you have an interest in anal play, get ready to dive into the donut hole with these techniques to access the ass.

Entering the Ass

Whether you want to proceed to anal penetration or just keep it light, you'll need to start with the anal basics. No matter what bits you're rocking, the anus and anal canal, "external" and "internal" sphincters, have a clever set of muscles that work hard to keep things like gas and bowel movements in until they are ready to be released, and once that time comes, the ass knows how to relax and open up. The same applies to backdoor lovin'. When the relaxation happens, many people find anal play to be extremely pleasurable, even transcendent at times. As a pirate would say, "Booty marks the spot on the pleasure map!"

How do you begin to warm up and relax the ass? First, as sex-ed Renaissance man Kenneth Play emphasizes, start by connecting with the human attached to the ass. Help them feel safe, calm, and aroused. It's crucial for the receiver of anal touch or penetration to be in their arousal beforehand. In other words, foreplay must come *first*. This can include the words you say to one another, the emotional connection you share, the kissing and touching of non-erogenous zones, hands-on genital or oral sex, using sex toys, spanking, flogging, or anything you're into. The key is to get into that arousal before getting into that ass. Once all parties, especially the receiver, are in their arousal state and have a full yes to experimenting with anal play, you can then implement these basics.

 Hack your way into anal artistry with episode #286, "A Sex Hackers' Guide to Anal Sex—with Kenneth Play."

Shameless Sex's Booty Basics

1. **Use lube.** Always use lube, and make sure it's thick and long-lasting. This is where silicone lubricants are extra beneficial, because they don't get absorbed into the skin the way water-based lubricants do. Überlube is top-notch for anal. If you're a die-hard water-based lube fan, then get a thicker gel formula like Sliquid's Sassy.

2. **Go slow—really slow.** Always start by going slow and taking your time. The booty will open when it's ready. Do *not* force anything into the ass, or any orifice for that matter, until that part of the body is ready for more. You can only make an exception to this if your partner is already super turned-on and screaming, "I want you in my ass now!" If this is the case, it could be a good time to speed things up. But no matter what, remember that any insertion into an unprepped and unrelaxed ass will take time.

3. **Start small.** Consider using one well-lubed finger to gently massage and rub the anal opening. If your partner feels ready (you can ask: "Are you ready for a finger?"), start by ever-so-lightly inserting one finger through the anus and into the anal canal. "Ever-so-lightly" means going slowly and barely pressing at all. Wait for the sensation of the ass opening and inviting you in. It's like waiting for the door to open after pressing the doorbell. Patience is key.

4. **You're in!** Once inside, hang out and relax for a minute and barely move that finger. Let the anal canal acclimate to it. Then, when it comes time to move your finger, move slower than slow and in a circular motion. Do *not* move your finger in and out because if you take your finger (or whatever is in the ass) out before the anal canal is fully relaxed, the gentle insertion process may need to start all over again. That slow circular motion can help further relax the sphincter muscles, which could lead to adding another finger. If you want to add another finger, do not pull the inserted finger out entirely. Instead, try sliding the second finger on top of the first finger while finger #1 remains inside the booty.

Full-on Anal Penetration

If you're interested in moving on to penetration after this warm-up, try letting the person receiving penetration be in control. One way to give the receiver control—after the anus and anal canal are relaxed and warmed up, of course—is for the receiver to squat or sit on the penetrating phallus. This allows the receiver to move at their own pace and take their time listening to their body. It might take thirty seconds, a few minutes, or it may just slip right in, but the key is for the receiver to accept the penetration in a way that is not overwhelming or painful.

If the receiver is wanting that cock or dildo in but it's just not happening, add more lube and bear down. Bearing down is when you internally push the pelvic floor muscles downward, like you're trying to push the penetrating object out. This may sound counterintuitive, but it actually helps open the sphincter muscles.

Want to add some consensual power play into the mix? If you're receiving while on top in a missionary position, and you feel your partner trying to move or thrust into you before your anus is a go, playfully but powerfully push down on their chest and say: *Don't move until I say move.* Not only will this serve as a reminder that you need more time while your body warms up, but it also adds an extra sense of hot dominance to the experience. Make sure your partner is okay with that kind of interaction first, though, because power play is not for everyone.

If the receiver is taking a long time to relax enough to be penetrated, and they're being penetrated by a penis, it's possible for the penis to start losing blood flow and the erection to subside. But never fear because hands and mouths are here! Use them to stimulate other areas of the body during the session. Kissing, nipple play, massaging the testicles, even taking two fingers around the cock at the base of the shaft while the head is making its way into the anus—all these actions can help maintain arousal during the experience.

Anal Pain Versus Discomfort

As you experiment with anal play, you may experience discomfort or pain. It's important to distinguish between these. Pain may feel like something burning or tearing and can possibly feel unbearable. Discomfort, however, is different from pain. When it comes to relaxing the ass during penetration, discomfort is common until the muscles have fully adjusted. Discomfort usually feels like an intense pressure, which eventually subsides with enough slowness, lubrication, and long, deep breaths.

While discomfort is okay and even normal, pain can be a sign that something is wrong. If you ever feel pain during anal play, slow down, add more lube, or stop playing all together. *Shameless Sex* **never** suggests using any sort of numbing agents for anal sex. That's a **hard no** to desensitizing the anus because it's important to stay aware of your body in case you're pushing beyond your body's tolerance level.

So don't get irritated at your discomfort (or pain); it's trying to tell you something. And when the discomfort dissipates, the back door is open for all kinds of ass play like moving with more speed, varying your movements, such as in-and-out thrusting, as well as switching up positions and angles.

Anal Toy How-Tos

Another way to both pleasure and relax the ass is through anal-safe sex toys. "Anal-safe" means there is a flared base preventing the toy from going all the way inside of the body (think of how the plastic part of a pacifier prevents choking). This is important because, unlike the vaginal canal, the ass does not have an ending. The anus leads to the anal canal, and then the anal canal opens to the rectum, and the rectum is connected to the colon and intestines and the rest of your body.

"Anal-safe" also means you're using toys that are nonporous so you can fully sanitize them after each use (and you should, because there's poop and bacteria that comes out of the ass). Look for toys made from medical-grade silicone or stainless steel.

Some of *Shameless Sex's* favorite anal toys include:

- **Butt plugs:** Butt plugs are great at relaxing the sphincter muscles and add a nice feeling of pressure. If you're a vulva owner, plugs can add compression to your vaginal canal, making stimulation of the G-area more pleasurable and even more accessible. Fun Factory makes a great set of plugs called the Bootie Plugs, and they come in three different sizes. If stainless-steel tickles your fancy, then Pure Plugs by Njoy are awesome for tapping that ass.
- **Anal beads:** At first glance, anal beads may be intimidating. Imagining a long rope of round balls inserted into your ass may seem like a lot to take in, but keep in mind that the anal canal is long and curvy and can handle much more than you may think. Using anal beads is not as much about the sensation of having them inside as it is about

the amazing feeling of slowly taking them out of the booty, before or during orgasm. If you want to explore anal beads but are intimidated by their length, start by inserting two to four of the beads and work your way up from there. Try a version made entirely of silicone so it's flexible and won't harbor bacteria.

- **Vibrating anal toys:** Anal pleasure is often about the physical pressure applied, as the internal anatomy of the ass doesn't have a lot of nerve endings to respond to vibrations. That's why a lot of butt plugs and anal beads don't vibrate. The anus, however, is packed with nerve endings, so vibrations can feel mind-blowing on this part of the external anatomy. Butt (wink wink) when going deeper inside to the anal canal, it's more about relaxation and pressure—and probably the taboo and naughtiness too. If you'd like to try a vibrating anal toy, remember to find one with a flared base. We love the PleX with Flex by Hot Octopuss because it has two motors that specifically target the external and internal parts of the ass.

That's just the tip of the anal iceberg. If you still want to expand your anal awareness, check out the multitude of *Shameless Sex* podcast episodes on this bootyful (and popular) topic. And if you're curious about prostate toys, including massagers, plugs, and harnesses, just keep reading because this back door discussion isn't done yet.

 Discover the perfect anal toys for *you* in episodes #118, "Sex Toys for Anal August," and #291, "2022's Top Sex Toys for Anal Play—with Amy and April."

Prostate Play How-Tos

What about playing with the prostate? The prostate is located inside the bodies of penis owners between the bladder and rectum and is best accessed through anal penetration (see diagram on page 239 for reference). It's embryologically similar to the G-area but is "deeper" inside the body. Therefore, the toys specifically designed for prostate stimulation are usually longer than your average butt plug. They also have an asymmetrical shape and curvature because the prostate is located on the anterior wall of the rectum (toward the belly button). If you're using fingers, it could take your longest finger to find it, and much like the G-area, it requires a curved "come hither" motion.

When accessing the prostate, the same booty basics apply, but now you're focusing on a specific type of pleasure and part of the body. Whether you're trying to discover your own prostate or you want to know how to pleasure a partner's prostate, go into it with low expectations the first time around because it takes time and practice. The location of the prostate varies from person to person, and it's not easy to distinguish which part of the rectum is actually prostate tissue. However, it's not completely indistinguishable either. *The Ultimate Guide to Prostate Pleasure* by Charlie Glickman, PhD, and Aislinn Emirzian reveals that the prostate has similar firmness to the tip of your nose, with a little indentation or crevice, while the rest of the rectum feels more like the softness of your cheek. During periods of heightened arousal, the prostate often becomes engorged and can become more noticeable to the touch.

Although prostate pleasure can be the star of the show, many people like to receive added stimulation on the penis, testicles, or other erogenous zones at the same time. Whether you're integrating other parts of the body or not, prostate stimulation can lead to more intense, full-bodied orgasms. As described by prostate toy developer and designer Forrest Andrews, many penis owners who have added prostate play to their sex lives reported having "super orgasms" beyond what they'd ever dreamed of.

And that's not all. *The Ultimate Guide to Prostate Pleasure* highlights that prostate play has benefits beyond just pleasure. Although research is limited, numerous studies suggest prostate stimulation may be linked to improved prostate health. These researchers and prostate aficionados believe regular prostate massage can potentially reduce age-related prostate issues, such as inflammation and enlargement. So, if you're looking to add a new item to your sexual menu, prostate play might be a healthy choice.

 Uncover the power of the prostate in episodes #11, "Prostate Pleasure and Health—with Charlie Glickman, PhD," and #298, "Prostates and Super Orgasms (and Enemas!)—with Forrest Andrews."

Pegging 101

Pegging is when a vulva owner penetrates the anus of their partner with a strap-on dildo. Though the anatomy and functions of the ass are similar no matter what genitals you're rocking, penis owners have that magical walnut-sized pleasure button residing in their asses (aka the prostate), so why not try and tap into it or least add it to your maybe list? While pegging is a widely misunderstood practice, there are still a ton of penis owners who love being pegged because there's nothing wrong with wanting to get fucked in the ass! Plus, it can be a lot of fun and arousing for the giver too.

 Strengthen your strap-on skills in episode #210, "Strap-On Sex 101—with Rain DeGrey."

If you're interested in pegging and you don't have a penis, here are a few product tips you might need (as a bonus, these can also apply to people without penises looking to strap it on with their partners during vaginal sex).

First of all, you'll need a harness. If you're a first-timer and don't want to spend too much cash, basic nylon-meets-plastic starter harnesses are a good option. However, they're often missing at least one of the key features you want in a quality harness. The first is for it to feel good and comfortable on your body. Second, it's ideal for the harness to have a strong hold so it can keep the dildo in place as you move your body. Third, you probably want to look and feel damn good in that harness. And fourth, look for a material that's easy to clean. Leather, for example, looks sexy when strapped on and can hold a dildo in place, but it's a porous material and thus more challenging to clean. Your best bet is to find a harness that has as many of those four aspects as possible, but understand that it may not hit all of them.

Once you've chosen your ideal harness, it's time to find a dildo that works for both you and your partner. Currently, the FDA (US Food and Drug Administration) does not regulate sex toys. The best way to tell if a toy is non-toxic is to shop at a sex-positive adult store and ask a staff member to guide you to the high quality, non-toxic items (if your're shopping online, ask via email). Also, if you can, give the toy a sniff test because non-toxic toys should *not* have a chemical smell.

Another important pegging consideration is finding the right size, shape, and color dildo. This is a great time to check in with your partner as to what kind of toy they want to be penetrated with. Also ask yourself what type of toy you feel comfortable and confident in strapping on: Do you want a dildo that looks realistic, with flesh tones and veins? Or do you prefer something that is good for penetration but does not look like an actual human body part? Do you want something specifically for prostate play, or do you want a universal toy with a more tapered tip that can be used for vaginal and anal play too? No matter what you choose, make sure the dildo has a base so it can stay in place in the harness.

Don't forget that dildos have a fixed size and shape, unlike real human body parts. While some have a softer, squishier texture allowing for better flexibity during penetration, many are made of firm silicone material. This is where size really does matter. Buy something a notch below the size that seems ideal to you—or better yet, ask your partner to choose the dildo because they know their body better than anyone else.

Once you've successfully found your ideal harness and dildo, the next question is: *What the fuck are you supposed to do with it?* When it comes to strap-on sex, it depends on what your partner(s) want and don't want. When you take on new variations of sex, have conversations beforehand and talk about boundaries, expectations, and needs. Plan what to do if things feel too intense, weird, or clunky. There is a high possibility that a non-penis owner with a silicone cock attached to their body will feel a bit out of their element—after all, this is a new experience! The more preliminary discussion, the better.

Creating safe words or signals for when things are feeling too uncomfortable or intense is a *must*. Also, coming to a common understanding of how to embrace the awkward is crucial. Welcome laughter when the dildo isn't hitting the right spot or your body feels clumsy because it's learning new ways to move and play. Remember that sex is called "play" for a reason, and embracing laughter and silliness can be a great addition to your sexy session.

Sacred Sexuality

Sex and intimacy can reach a new level of profound connection, love, healing, and mind-blowing (even soul-shaking) pleasure when combined with spirituality. "Sacred sexuality" is an umbrella term that covers a wide range of methodologies and practices that link sex and intimacy with spirituality. Spirituality in this context does not necessarily refer to religion, although if you want to declare your sacred sex practice as part of your religion, then more power to you. In a sexual context, spirituality means different things for everyone. It could be a feeling that the sex you're having connects you with something beyond yourself, such as divinity, the universe, a source, spirit, or a sense of oneness. For many, sacred sexuality leads to a sense of wholeness and a deepened union with their partner(s).

For a lot of folks, sacred sexuality can seem intimidating. Amy used to be one of those people. Although she saw the potential for deeper connection with a partner through Tantra, she had never experienced sex in that way. Sex, to her, was always a physical exchange of pleasure between two separate bodies. She could easily relate to sex that resembled "fucking," but the idea of experiencing oneness during sex while going slow or "making love" seemed unattainable for her. However, one night in a Las Vegas hotel room with a lover, sacred sexuality *found her* unexpectedly, and it transformed her perspective.

While Amy and her lover had never engaged in sexual touch before this life-changing evening, they did spend months getting to know each other through continuous flirtation. So when it felt right to explore skin-on-skin contact, they agreed to implement the same slow reverence, making boundaries and safety a top priority. Genitals were off the table, and both of them remained fully clothed because the engagement was less about sex and more about sensuality and connection. From deep eye-gazing to fingers slowly trickling down her arms and legs, to lips on exposed skin, their bodies moved and rubbed against each other like an erotic dance. Amy felt like she had blasted off into a whole different world where two bodies merged into one, vibrating in a timeless vortex of sensual pleasure.

As Amy's story illustrates, sacred sexuality is more about presence and connection than sex and orgasms. The key is to create an intentional container where all parties not only feel respected and cared for, but they're also revered. Sacred sexuality is an opportunity to take eroticism to new heights by inviting in a sense of mutual honoring, worshiping, and adoration. How you decide to incorporate it into your life is up to you. Some form of sacred sexuality is obtainable for all people, and it can be a lifestyle, a daily practice, a hobby, or something you tap into from time to time.

In fact, many experts have spent decades researching, refining, and evolving the variations of sacred sexuality and how they may apply to different people. Neotantra is one of these variations. It is similar to what most of the Western world knows as Tantra, though that sexual aspect is just a tiny piece of a very large puzzle. Tantra is an ancient spiritual practice originating in India that involves presence, reverence, and ritual far beyond sensual or sexual connection with others. Neotantra and other sacred sexualities can help expand familiar or routine sex further than the physical and into a transcendental world of infinite possibilities.

Barbara Carrellas, world-renowned teacher of Neotantra, also links Tantric sex to kink and BDSM play, highlighting the unlimited opportunities for adding the sacred into your sexual play. The feeling of oneness Tantric sex provides can serve as a sexy safety bubble for consensual kink exploration. In her book *Urban Tantra: Sacred Sex for the Twenty-First Century*, Carrellas explains that BDSM itself can be a form of sacred sexuality.

 Tantalize yourself with Tantra in episode #257, "How to Have Energy Orgasms—with Barbara Carellas."

Spanking of BDSM (whoops, we meant "speaking of")—grab your floggers and paddles because it's time to explore the thrilling world of kink.

Kink and BDSM

"Kink" is another blanket term that encompasses countless types of sexual exploration. Kink educator and expert Orpheus Black defines it simply: "Kink is any deviation from what you think is normal sexual behavior. What's important about this is it's any deviation from what *you* think. Not what your friend thinks or what the television thinks or what porn thinks. It's any deviation from what *you* think is . . . normal sexual behavior."

As Orpheus Black emphasizes, what counts as "deviating from the norm" will differ from person to person and place to place and will shift as time goes on. You don't need a dungeon, ball gag, paddles, or a bunch of leather to be kinky; the definition and experience is entirely up to you and anyone you play with. That being said, there are a few key points to keep in mind if you're pursuing kinky play.

 Master the art of safe, sexy, and consensual BDSM in episodes #243, "How to Be More Dominant in the Bedroom (for Penis Owners)," #267, "Spank Me! Choke Me! (but learn these tools first)," and #278, "The Submissive Side of BDSM—with Orpheus Black."

First, as Orpheus Black also stresses, it's important to do as much research as possible before entering into potentially intense sexual experiences. Playing with kink and BDSM can be incredibly hot and satisfying, but it requires a considerable amount of education to get to those places. Commit to always learning. If you're interested in kink courses or personal coaching sessions and seminars, check out the work of sexologist and kink educator Orpheus Black, or Sunny Megatron, or Jaeleen Bennis and Eve Minax, co-authors of *Bondassage: Kinky Erotic Massage Tips for Lovers.*

 Continue your kink education with episodes #246, How to Do Kink and Erotic Play Your Way—with Sunny Megatron," #58, "Bondassage—with Jaeleen Bennis," and #159, "Kink and BDSM In Relationships—with Eve Minax."

In kink as well as any other form of sex or sexual touch, make sure that you're obtaining full active consent from all parties involved. When it comes to riskier explorations such as BDSM, it's crucial to have your consent game down. This includes understanding what consent means, the art of negotiation, and being proactive about implementing, conveying, and listening to boundaries.

Next up are communication skills. These are important in all aspects of sex and relationships, but when it comes to kink, they're **nonnegotiable**. Communication can be with or without words, but all parties need to know how to communicate and understand when something is too much. This includes everything from: "When I say stop, I mean stop" to "Sometimes I say stop but I don't really want to stop, so if I say red that means stop" to "When it's hard for me to speak up or our play makes it difficult for me to speak, I'll tap you three times if I want you to stop what you're doing," and so on. Safe words can come in all different forms, and it's important to talk about them *before* entering a potentially risky experience.

Last but not least, don't forget to finish any highly intense sexual experiences with aftercare. Aftercare needs vary from person to person and even within the same person over time. An individual's ideal aftercare could range from being gently held and touched to having vocal conversations about the experience. What felt good? What felt a bit edgy? What leaned a bit too close to a hard no? What needs to shift for future explorations to become even better? Like other aspects of communication, it's helpful to discuss aftercare needs *before* entering a highly intense sexual space. Initiate discussions about what all parties are desiring to happen during and after playtime *beforehand.* This doesn't prevent harm, miscommunication, or missteps from happening, but it makes them much less probable.

Role-Play

In Chapter 3 you learned the distinction between fantasies that are meant to reside in the internal spank bank versus those that you may want to act out in real life. Amy's fantasies of sexual violence and April's stepparent fantasy are great examples of fantasies that didn't represent our actual desires, but did point us in the direction of things that interested us, like dominance and submission.

When everyone is on board and open to it, discussing your fantasies can be a sexy, arousing, and a fun experience. If you find yourself in this place, it's a great time to revisit (or create) your list of yeses and maybes and compare it with your partner's list to see what aligns. Once you have a better understanding of how you can lean into each other, start thinking about what these scenarios might look like. For example, if you have a fantasy about being a doctor whose patient seduces you in the exam room, and your partner is a yes to taking this fantasy into role-play, what do you both envision this scene to look like? Collaborate on the details. Are you wearing a lab coat and stethoscope? Why is your patient in the exam room in the first place? And once they seduce you, what happens next? Are you having sex on the exam table? If so, what kind of sex? Get clear about what's on and off the table (literally and figuratively).

Remember that when it comes to bringing fantasy into real life, what you've seen in porn or envisioned in your mind will probably be very different from the actual live experience. Again, this is why sex is referred to as play! If the scenario you thought would be a mega turn-on starts to feel awkward or silly, just have fun with it. It's okay to go from being the confident, powerful, sexy doctor wearing a lab coat to the goofy person who doesn't know what to do next. Speak to it, laugh about it, and take a few deep breaths, then jump back into the role. And if you're feeling like you want to change or stop the experience altogether, that's okay too. Just cross that item off your sexy to-do list and then pat yourself on the back because you just learned more about your sexuality.

 Learn how to have fun with roleplay in episode #97, "Role-Play and How to Be Dominant in the Bedroom— with Midori."

The Raw and Rewarding World of Threesomes

According to *Shameless Sex*'s listener questions and the number of episode downloads, threesomes are a very popular and common fantasy for a lot of people, regardless of their relationship status or style. There are many reasons why having a threesome is so attractive. It's been sensationalized in porn and media, and it's perceived as somewhat acceptable within the societal norms of mainstream monogamy. For those in a committed relationship, a threesome can sound like a safe, exciting way to explore opening the relationship, since both parties get to participate. And for others, the idea of having sex with more than one person just sounds hot regardless of the relationship style they're in.

However, not to burst your bubble, threesomes are *not* always as satisfying or as easy as they may seem. As Dr. Lori Beth Bisbey explains, when you add more than one person to your playtime, you're also adding another individual with their own set of emotional and physical needs. If you struggle relating to the needs of one partner, imagine trying to navigate the differing erotic landscapes of two partners. There's also the risk of someone feeling left out. Because of this, Dr. Bisbey suggests playing in even numbers, like in a foursome. That way, if two people click and are connecting deeply, the other two can focus on each other and still have fun without feeling excluded, leaving less potential for hurt to arise.

 Dip your toes into threesomes with episodes #72, "Threesome Stories and Tips—with Amy and April," and #277, "How to Add More Hotness and Desire in Your Relationship—with Dr. Lori Beth Bisbey."

Threesome How-Tos

As stated throughout this chapter, it's important to take the time to educate yourself about any unfamiliar sexual practices before hopping right in—especially when it comes to riskier explorations where safety is involved or feelings can get hurt. While some people are fortunate enough to have a magical, amazing threesome where everyone leaves completely joyful and satisfied despite little to no conversation preceding the experience (as seen in porn), this is not how it will usually go. As Reid Mihalko, sex educator and threesome expert, puts it, "A porn threesome is an actual threesome, but it's a threesome with Olympic athletes of sexuality. And for those of us who are not Olympic athletes, who are just amateurs, it's a little clunkier." But, he says, "[it] can still be just as fun. Getting a bunch of your musician friends together to play Van Halen might not exactly sound like Van Halen playing Van Halen, but it still can be damn fun!"

In order have some damn fun in a threesome, it's *incredibly* important to initiate conversations about needs and desires *before* the sexual action takes place because entering with unspoken hopes or assumptions can lead to a (preventable) mess. Mihalko says, "Understand that when you invite somebody to have a threesome, they might be thinking double penetration and all the things they've seen in porn—meanwhile your vision of a threesome is the three of you taking a shower together and making out. . . So, understanding and having a conversation about what a successful threesome means for you and what it means for everybody else, along with understanding what would not be successful, is really important. This means having a conversation about expectations, not about what we have to do but more about what we're wanting and how we know if this went well."

Aside from hopes and expectations, what about boundaries? What feels like a yes, a maybe, and a hard no? This is where the practice of creating and then combining your sexual menus will again be very effective.

Talk about the key pieces: *Where do we align, and what is on and off the table right now? What happens if someone starts to feel uncomfortable? How will they let everyone know? What happens if feelings change in the moment and something goes beyond our combined yes and maybe lists? Or what happens if we want to slow down or stop whatever we thought we were both into ahead of time?*

Once you and your partner have clarified your combined intentions, then it's time to expand into your vision for the third person involved. Consider all the elements: Are you looking for a penis-owning third, vulva-owning third, or are you open to whomever? What are the qualities of this other person? Is this someone you've already met, like an acquaintance or close friend? Does it feel like a safer choice to engage with a third who is not a part of your community or lives in a different zip code? If all goes well, is the option to play again on the table or is this just a one-time exploration? And what if one of you connects with the third and the other one doesn't? How will you navigate this space?

Especially for couples who are brand-new to exploring threesomes, it's important to remember that the third party (the rare and highly coveted "unicorn") will have their own set of wants and needs that deserve to be considered equally to yours. After all, they're a person too, and if you intend to invite them into your erotic container, treat them with respect and consideration. Have another deep conversation (or two) about everyone's desires, needs, and boundaries once you've found your unicorn. Mihalko explains, "Threesomes can be really activity-based for people as opposed to people-based, and for some, threesomes can be more feelings-based rather than activity-based. Prior negotiation [of all activities is crucial], [as is being] able to check in, navigate, and follow the flow of where things are going along the way." Communicating clearly also gives your unicorn autonomy in their choice to play with you. This conversation should include a discussion about safer sex as well, especially if touching genitals or sharing fluids is on the menu. (To learn how to easily do this, go back to page 77 in Chapter 2 for Mihalko's "Safer-Sex Elevator Speech.") You, your partner, and your unicorn all deserve the opportunity to both express and hear clear sexual expectations and boundaries within a safe environment.

For example, maybe you and your partner decide this is a one-time thing, and your partner gets to give and receive with the third with mouths, fingers, and gyrating bodies, and the boundaries of your participation are that you can engage in the initial kissing and heavy petting on non-genital parts of the body, but you back off and only watch when your partner gives you the signal. Be clear about this with whomever you're inviting for the threesome beforehand. Also decide what happens afterward. Do you all drink a cup of tea together and talk about it? Do you have a snuggly slumber party? What does everyone need for aftercare, so things feel good before going your separate ways? Mihalko shares his approach on threesomes: "When I see people after we've had a threesome, I don't want to wonder if it's going to be awkward because people have regrets or feel weird about it . . . Even if we never have another threesome together again, I want people to feel good they did whatever they did with me."

Mihalko recommends not setting the bar too high at the very beginning. Start slow, especially if this is new to you. "Slow" varies from person to person, so if your concept of slow means exploring with kissing and non-genital touch all over the body, then do that. In Mihalko's view, "If all three people are going to have a threesome and this is everyone's first threesome . . . all parties . . . should probably go really slow, so they're sure they do a good job with each other." After all, it's easier to check in along the way as opposed to moving quickly and hurting or triggering someone in your rush. Being slow and considerate can also mean waiting until future sessions to explore further. As Mihalko puts it, "If the spontaneous organic threesome everyone dreams of is on the table, let that be the fifth time you all get together."

As you go, remember to stay present and be aware of what's going on with the people around you. Mihalko adds, "No matter how many times you've hooked up with people (and especially if it's the first time you're hooking up), pay attention to everybody and where they're at. Everyone is going to be in different places from moment to moment. The more mindful you can be to those nuances, hopefully the safer everyone will feel when all parties communicate in more explicit ways." This can be especially helpful if voicing boundaries in the heat of the moment is difficult for you. If you're concerned (or if you just want to be prepared), be sure to let your play partners know how to look out for your nonverbal signals beforehand and ask them about theirs. As Mihalko says, "When you're paying attention to soft nos and body language of the people you're playing with, these things help create environments that foster positive outcomes rather than missed opportunities or messy situations," no matter what kind of sex you're having.

It's also important to remember that it's 100 percent okay to try something and then change your mind—this is a process of exploring, after all. If you find yourself feeling a "no" or even an "I don't know but this doesn't feel that great," press pause and take time to tend to your needs.

Your partners wouldn't want you leaving with a not-so-great feeling, just like you wouldn't want that for them either. When your partner voices their needs, listen and thank them for their honesty and being clear with you. People are often hesitant to express their boundaries about their sex lives, so it's crucial to offer positive reinforcement when they do. This will help ensure they continue to feel comfortable speaking up in the future.

If you're feeling exhausted by the extreme emphasis on communication before, during, and after new sexual experiences, it may be a good idea to delay any plans for a threesome until you've taken the time for some personal exploration and growth. Sometimes threesomes are meant to remain a fantasy, and that's okay. But if you have the willingness to work on refining your sexual communication skills, then you're setting the stage for a positive threesome experience for everyone.

 Take an even deeper dive into the world of threesomes in episode #105, "Threesomes—with Reid Mihalko."

Where Is the Unicorn?

If you're wondering where to find that third person to play with or how to become the unicorn third for a couple, you're not alone. Unfortunately, there are no tried-and-true instructions for this because it all depends on location, access, and preference. Dating apps are a great place to start, and some are more geared toward openness around sexuality, like Feeld.co. Many people seeking out a threesome create a profile clearly stating in their bio what they're looking for. Some couples create a combined profile, while others make individual profiles but maintain transparency about their relationship status and their desire for a third. If you're interested in becoming a unicorn, you can specify that on your profile or in the online chat exchanges with other couples. The demand is higher than the supply, so you'll probably be highly coveted and sought after, just like a mythological unicorn.

There are also retreats and resorts (often called "lifestyle resorts") that cater to nonmonogamous explorations, primarily centered around the world of swinging, where couples swap partners or play with each other. There are also plenty of threesomes, foursomes, and orgies that take place at these resorts. Most are located in warm climates and are on tropical islands or cruise ships and can be found in many parts of the world. So if a swingers' resort is intriguing to you and within your budget, do your research and see what offerings resonate with you most.

If you're fortunate enough to find your unicorn, remember that they are a human being and are as much a part of the experience as you and your partner. Mihalko suggests checking in and thanking them afterward. This could be done through a text message, a phone call, or even an email saying something like: *Hey, you. Last night was really fun. Thank you for playing with us/me. I/we also wanted to check in to see how you're feeling about last night and if there's anything you're needing from us/me. I/we want you to feel cared for because I/we appreciate you and enjoyed our time together.* This is part of being a considerate sexually explorative human. And, if you have intentions of playing with this person again, it might work in your favor for securing those future endeavors.

There are also entire books dedicated to refining the art of threesomes, such as *The Ultimate Guide to Threesomes* by author and sex and intimacy coach Stella Harris. Remember, through continuous education, practice, and communication, you will likely have a much higher return on your three-way investment and ensure more positive intimate experiences in the future.

 For another in-depth perspective on threesomes, check out episode #211, "The Ultimate Guide to Threesomes— with Stella Harris."

I DON'T KNOW HOW TO KEEP SEX HOT AND CONNECTED AFTER PHYSIOLOGICAL SHIFTS

My partner was diagnosed with a major physiological health condition in childhood and just recently had surgery, resulting in chronic pain and limiting certain sex positions. I love my partner, and I'm 1,000 percent on board with finding new ways to have sex without causing them more pain. We have open communication where they have shared what feels good and what doesn't anymore since the surgery, but I'm curious if there are better ways I can support my partner and our relationship so we can stay intimately connected and continue to have hot sex.

Chapter 1 covered how to handle significant changes in sexuality by looking at the psychological factors involved with sex (such as performance and arousal). Chapter 2 went deeper into the mental and emotional shifts that can occur when someone's experience of sexuality takes an unexpected turn, while touching on the physiological shifts as well (such as aging, trauma, and getting an STI). This section offers a deeper dive into how to navigate physiological shifts when they happen—but with a spicy emphasis on bringing newness, excitement, and passion into the bedroom when living with a disability.

As award-winning disability awareness consultant Andrew Gurza's work affirms, individuals living with a disability or undergoing major life changes can still experience or re-create sexiness in countless ways. Add to that supportive partners who are eager to learn how to keep the spark alive and the sex connected, and the potential for intimacy and pleasure is limitless. Whether you're personally navigating changes in your physical experience of sex or supporting a partner through their journey, it's time to take things up a notch and CYOPP to find your way to pleasure town.

 Learn how to have hot sex with disabilities in episode #103, "Sex, Disability, and Disabled People Are Hot—with Andrew Gurza."

I DON'T KNOW HOW TO KEEP SEX HOT AND CONNECTED AFTER PHYSIOLOGICAL SHIFTS

1. Do you want to gain more awareness around your partner's experience of disability and sex as well as learn how to be a more supportive partner in the bedroom? If so, continue to read this chapter.

2. Would you like to expand your erotic menu with new techniques and positions specifically geared toward more pleasure and physical comfort for your partner who's living with a disability? If so, continue to read this chapter.

3. Do you want to discover the many options available when it comes to finding new ways to play? If so, continue to read this chapter for items you can add to your sexual menu. We also recommend going back to pages 88 and 89 of **Chapter 2: Am I Broken?** for a variety of ideas to reinvent sex with your partner.

How to Be a Supportive Partner Through Life's Changes

Having a partner living with chronic pain or disability, as well as any other significant life changes, can be challenging. Your partner probably has their own set of frustrations due to the limitations encompassing these shifts, and if that's not hard enough, they're also experiencing the physical toll of chronic pain every single day. With that said, it might be time to seek outside support to gain a better understanding of your partner's experience, especially if this situation is new to you.

Consulting a therapist specializing in chronic pain (or other trained professional) can help you further comprehend what your partner is going through and figure out how to work with it. As Dr. Lee Phillips, certified sex and couple's therapist specializing in chronic illness and sexuality, explains, "Many people living with disability or chronic pain . . . tend to think of themselves as their condition. That's something I work on with individuals and couples: You are not your illness. It's a part of you, but we should focus on what you can do, and when it comes to sex, let's consider what's achievable rather than what used to be possible." He adds, "My patients usually say, 'Wait, I can be sexual? I can be touched in new ways?' Understanding and accepting this is the key to getting through [this major life change] and to rediscovering pleasure." There are so many options to explore and add to your combined sexual menus, so why not focus on those?

Introducing the Idea of Seeking Outside Support (and Finding the Right Therapist)

In Chapter 2, we talked about how you can't force someone to go to therapy or work on themselves. However, you can lovingly ask your partner to join you in seeking a therapist together—maybe just for a few sessions to start. Emphasize how it can be a shared exploration that will benefit everyone involved. If you get a yes from your partner and they agree to take this journey with you, be sure to find a qualified therapist who not only specializes in your specific needs but is also someone all parties feel safe and secure with.

When trying to find the right therapist, it's important to do your homework. Start by making a list of potential candidates, and then scour their online presence to get a sense of their approach to therapy. Investigate with your partner and discuss who seems like the best fit. Once you've narrowed down your options, reach out to set up a session or consultation. Keep in mind that not all therapists may be taking new clients, so don't be discouraged if your top choices are fully booked months in advance or unable to work with you. Keep searching because with persistence, the right support system will come your way.

Each of your own unique sets of desires and needs should be taken into account throughout the process. When supporting a partner with a disability, particularly a recent one, you'll have to be aware of what Dr. Phillips calls "the caregiving stress syndrome," when the lines between partner and caregiver are blurred. "When a chronic illness is encountered in a partnership, it can be life-changing," he remarks. But it's okay to have complex emotions. According to Dr. Phillips, "At the start of a chronic illness, there is often a period of crisis. There is a rupture in the relationship often leading to a lack of sexual desire." If this is relatable to you, it doesn't mean that something is wrong with your relationship; it just means that you need time to adjust to the situation.

Change is an inevitable component in all relationships. According to Dr. Phillips, no matter if one partner has a chronic illness, disability, or not, bodies and connections evolve as time passes. The same goes for sex. But if you treat each other's requirements—physical or emotional—with "trust, honesty, communication, and respect," then your relationship can continue to develop positively.

Especially in the realm of sex, empathy and communication are absolutely essential. Dr. Phillips points out that people tend to assume they know what their partner wants—but they forget that things can change with time. That's why it's important to talk about sex and intimacy on a regular basis. If that seems difficult, then find a therapist that meets your specific needs so you can work together to address the issues. They can guide the discussion so everyone can better express themselves in an understandable way. Dr. Phillips often asks questions including, "What was your sex like before the illness? Were you having sex, and what type of sex were you having? Also, what does sex mean to you?" He emphasizes learning how to express your needs and then continuously practicing with your partner.

Both your and your partner's needs are valid, and you'll share the goal of working together to find a better understanding of each other's changing bodies. This will take communication skills and openness to exploring and experimenting with new sexual options, including things like new positions, nonsexual touch, sexual touch minus penetration, sex toys, finding other outlets for getting certain needs met, and so much more. The good news is your experimentation can also be fun! We encourage you to approach experimentation as more of a lifestyle as opposed to a phase, because ultimately this is what having a hotter, steamier, more connected sex life is all about. It's completely up to you which direction you take, but keep in mind that a whole buffet of options is available to help you create an entirely new and delectable sexual menu.

 Find ways to keep the sexiness sizzling while living with chronic pain in episode #96, "Sex, Relationships, and Chronic Illness (and Pain)—with Dr. Lee Phillips."

Techniques for Turning Up the Heat

Like Dr. Phillips, Kelly Gordon, sex and disability expert and co-founder of the disability-inclusive recruitment agency With Not For, recommends thinking positively about "what you can and can't do. It's always best to be honest with yourself and your partner. It can still be sexy and hot when you talk about which positions work for you." Gordon shares some of her suggestions for the best sex positions that are friendlier to people with physical disabilities below.

- **Spooning.** This is great for any occasion. You can make it slow and tender *or* hard and fast. It's good for reserving energy levels while still maximizing pleasure during sexy time. This is a fabulous go-to in the mornings if you and your partner want a quickie before the kids wake up, or if you're looking for a lazy late-night session after a long day.
- **Collapsed doggy.** This is an amazing position for PIV sex when the penis owner has more mobility. The vulva owner lies flat on their stomach with their legs together, while the penis owner is on top and behind. This allows the receiver to enjoy doggy without worrying about maintaining an arched position.
- **Sex with pillows and straps.** These products can assist with different sex positions that might otherwise have been difficult, strenuous, or unachievable. Sportsheets and Liberator are just a few of the companies that make excellent straps and wedges that help support different areas of the body and are great for positioning. Some of these products even allow your partner to hold you up while you're in your sexual experience.

In addition to pillows and straps, incorporating sex toys can also be a game changer. If you're considering using toys, Gordon suggests thinking outside the box: "It's important to know just because something says it's an anal toy or a G-spot vibrator doesn't mean you have to use it in that particular way. Play around and figure out what works for you and your partner."

For penis owners with disabilities, both *Shameless Sex* and Gordon recommend Pulse Solo Interactive by Hot Octopuss. Not only can it be pleasurable whether you're flaccid or erect, but it can also be used completely hands-free. Plus, it can be controlled from a mobile phone (so your partner or long-distance lover can control your pleasure) and it syncs with online content so you "feel what you see."

For vulva owners, Gordon says to "get a good vibrating wand!" Wands are so versatile and usually have longer handles so they don't require a lot of reach. A wand that's packed with power is great for those days when you want to kick back, relax, and enjoy letting the toy do all the work. Also, most are so powerful that you can use them over your clothes and still feel the intensity, which is an added bonus when you're trying to relax and focus on your pleasure.

 Discover the right positions and toy for your body's unique needs in this bonus episode, "Pleasure Rebels, Hot Sex with Disabilities, & Sex Toys—with Kelly Gordon."

THE WORLD IS YOUR OYSTER

Regardless of your life circumstances and relationship status, it can be hard to make sure the bedroom remains a place of fun and excitement. Encourage curiosity about each other's desires and share them often. Be energetic and imaginative to make the most of every moment because you never know where the next adventure will take you. Plus, when you're equipped with openness and the willingness to try new sexual options to add to your sexual menu, the opportunities for finding new ways to play are limitless. From sex toys and positioning to communication techniques and experimenting with exciting newness, you have the power to thrive in the bedroom and ignite your sex life to keep it hot and full of passion. The world is your oyster—go ahead and grab that one-of-a-kind sexual pearl!

How Can I Keep the Fire Burning?

This final chapter is not the end, but the beginning to your sexual journey. It's all about integrating the valuable knowledge and skills you've acquired from this book into your life. Whether you're mastering the art of communication, prioritizing sexual self-care, refining your erotic techniques, or revisiting your sexual menu, frequent practice is an absolute *must* and the only way you will achieve the sex and relationship outcomes you desire. However, let's step away from the idea of "practice makes perfect." There is no such thing as "perfect" when it comes to pleasure. It's an ever-evolving journey with endless possibilities for growth and expansion. There is no final destination where the work is no longer needed. Instead, the consistent effort will move you toward greater heights of pleasure and fulfillment.

Your progress won't always be linear. Maybe you've done the work and grown beyond what you'd ever imagined, having great sex with yourself and your partner(s). But somewhere down the road, you hit a block. The sex dwindles, connection to your body and desire fades, or what once felt easy and exciting now seems challenging and misaligned, leaving you or your partner(s) confused, lost, and possibly disappointed. Breaking news: this is an inevitable part of being a human! Sex, along with almost every aspect of life on planet Earth, involves a constant ebb and flow. "Happily ever after" is an invention of fairy tales—and who knows what happened to those couples five years after the storybook wedding (hint: they experienced changes too)!

It's a well-known fact that the greatest of masters never stop learning. So even when you feel like you've become a master of your sex and relationships, that doesn't mean you're done learning. It's like tending to a fire: you have to keep adding fuel and stoking the flames. When something big changes in a relationship, it's an opportunity for personal inquiry and collaborative growth. This includes exploring how past experiences have influenced your connection to your present body, fine-tuning your communication skills, questioning old grudges and hang-ups, tackling those scary conversations about needs and fantasies, finding ways to connect intimately with your partner, and discovering new opportunities to make sex better beyond what you even imagined.

In other words, your sexual and relational journey often requires an openness to moving two steps forward and then one step back. To paraphrase bestselling author Dr. Brené Brown's notion of "perfectly imperfect," your imperfection is not a problem but instead an opportunity to reassess your situation and reimplement the tools you've learned again and again. It's okay to feel as though you've fallen off the horse and like you're "stuck" again. All you have to do is hop back on that pony, giddyup, and ride off into the sunset (to the sound of Leonard Cohen singing, "There is a crack, a crack in everything / That's how the light gets in.").

It's our ultimate desire that this book will serve as a go-to resource for you anytime you fall off that proverbial horse, need a boost of confidence, or just want a little bit of sexual inspiration. Always remember: no matter where you are on your journey, *Shameless Sex* will be here waiting for you, just like a big, warm hug.

PROACTIVE TOOLS TO KEEP YOUR OWN FIRE BURNING

Most people think about the roller coaster of sex and relationships as primarily centered in how you connect with others, but it's crucial to understand the importance of intimate connection with yourself too. This involves how you relate to your sex drive or body, as well as how you feel about your shifting needs. That said, we'd love to leave you with some final tips so you can continue proactively connecting with yourself and your desires.

1. **Never stop learning.** If you're a single person, keep absorbing information about sex and relationship skills on your own. If you're partnered, do so individually *and* with your partner(s). There are limitless online and in-person resources out there, such as sex-ed classes, workshops, podcasts, and audio and printed books, all of which will give you plenty of new ideas to keep things fresh. Better yet, once you've discovered something on your own, make sure to discuss it with your lover(s) too. That way everyone can learn, and they'll have a better idea of where you are on your sexual journey.

2. **Never stop batin'.** Speaking of learning about yourself . . . self-pleasure is imperative for staying connected to and reconnecting with your sexuality. Check in regularly to see what wants and needs are present or have shifted and how you can tend to your pleasure. The level of participation is entirely up to you—you can set aside time to masturbate every day, or you can simply think about it every once in a while, if that's more your speed. Both will earn you a *Shameless Sex* high five. However, the more time that passes where you're disconnected from your sexuality, the more time it will take to get reacquainted with it. So why not be proactive by staying attuned to your pleasure, just like you do with other aspects of your health and well-being?

3. **Never stop seducing . . . you!** It may seem simple, but another key part of staying connected with your sexuality is by loving yourself—and no, that's not a euphemism. There are many ways to exercise continuous self-love and self-acceptance. According to pleasure coach and author of *Slow Pleasure* Euphemia Russell, one way involves learning how to flirt . . . with yourself! Consider expressing adoration and appreciation for yourself the way you would for a lover. Stand in front of a mirror and remind yourself, verbally or nonverbally, how fucking fantastic you are. You can even add in a little seduction. Go ahead, hit on yourself over and over again—we dare you!

 Brush up on how to flirt with . . . *you* in episode #305, "How To Up Your Flirting Game—with Euphemia Russell."

4. **Never stop fueling your fire.** What makes you feel most alive in your being or good in your body? Is it getting out in nature, meditating, listening to beautiful music, or immersing yourself in embodied activities like dance, exercise, or other forms of movement? Perhaps it's starting a new creative project that fills you with purpose and excitement. Maybe it's spending quiet time with yourself while cozied up with a book. Or is it spending quality time with good friends—or putting those social-butterfly wings on and meeting new people? Whatever lights you up inside, do it often. The more light and joy there is in your life, the more there will be in your sex life.

AVOIDING GETTING STUCK IN A RUT AGAIN WITH PARTNERS

If you've read this book from cover to cover, then you probably already know how common it is for sex between partners to have highs and lows. Sometimes, people simply grow apart over time, especially when they come together without a well-defined understanding of their core values and sex and relationship needs. For others, a lack of communication can lead to shifts in the relationship. But even for well-matched partners with great communication, change is inevitable. The initial lust phase is bound to transform into something less consuming and more comfortable or even predictable. But through skilled, loving, and continuous communication, partners can work together to maintain their ever-evolving connection—potentially even making it stronger.

Consider the following recommendations to be the logs you can throw on your relational fire to keep the passion burning (or reignite it if it ever starts to dwindle).

1. **Embrace change.** Again, all sex and relationships change, and that's a fact! Most of the time, you'll be able to handle these changes, but some (like aging, trauma, and health issues) come with more challenges than others. If you feel like you're in misalignment, don't throw in the towel and cancel the relationship before you truly feel you've tried everything—including seeking outside support. Change is an opportunity to reevaluate what is true in your relationship now. By taking into consideration the shifts that have occurred, you can cultivate new relationship structures and ways to play that all parties can lean into.

2. **Be proactive.** Skilled relationship counselors Don and Martha Rosenthal advise "more truth sooner," meaning if you feel that there's a problem (or that things are okay but could be better), speak to it sooner than later. *Don't wait* for shit to hit the fan before you work on it or seek support. Being proactive about preventing problems is the key to unlocking a harmonious and loving (as well as a hot and intimate) relationship. Waiting until things get really bad, or until they go from bad to worse, will only lead to more time, more energy, and likely more money spent on repairing the damage.

3. **Cultivate connection.** One vital way to be proactive involves being intentional about setting aside time for your relationship. First, schedule regular check-ins at *least* once a month (but if you want

an A+ on your *Shameless Sex* report card, aim for at least once a week). A check-in is an opportunity for you and your partner to keep each other up to date on the current state of your union. Feel free to include anything regarding your relationship. Sex, touch, intimacy, love, connection, sexual menu items, communication, date nights, frustrations about the kids or the laundry—it's all related and real.

Check-ins may bring up resistance and fear because these conversations will not always be perfect. For more gentleness and ease, start your sex life check-in with the positives: *What's feeling good and working really well? What do I want more of and what are some ways I want to explore this with my partner?* Lastly, if applicable, lovingly bring up what's not working or feeling good and needs to be addressed as part of honoring your desires.

After you share, ask your partner about their own wants and desires, and actively listen to their responses. What feels good for them, what do they desire more of, and what doesn't align with their needs? It's important to stay curious about your partner's unique experience—the check-in is a two-way street.

It's also key to schedule regular date nights (or afternoons or sunrises) or intimate time together—ideally weekly. Intimacy date nights do *not* have to lead to sex. They're more about staying connected and understanding where each person is emotionally in that moment. To learn about variations of date nights (including "giving and receiving nights"), go back to Chapter 4.

4. **Spice it up.** Continue exploring newness within the boundaries of your relationship. This can be sexual—like spending an evening

slowly kissing and nibbling parts of your partner's body or going on a field trip to your local sex shop and then trying out your purchases—or it can just be about quality time. Things like surprising your partner by decorating the kitchen like a fancy restaurant for dinner or inviting them to a game night with just the two of you—these things count too! Sexual and otherwise, the possibilities are endless. The key here is to try new activities regularly, whether it's adding sex toys, trying kinky play, exploring some backdoor action, exchanging erotic fantasies with each other, or simply going for a walk while holding hands. For a refresher on newness, Chapter 7 has you covered.

To receive *Shameless Sex*'s curated list of over sixty fun and creative sexy things to do to spice things up with lovers, sign up for our newsletter at shamelesssex.com.

---

5. **Get unstuck with support.** If you're stuck to the point where you feel unable to move forward in your relationship, seek support! Find a reputable and unbiased third party to help you navigate your relational terrain. This does *not* mean you or your partner are weak or broken. In fact, seeking support is about the strongest, fiercest, and most proactive thing you can do in the bedroom and in life. There is a reason why people say, "Relationships take work," and this doesn't have to be a bad thing. It's part of accepting that humans have ever-changing minds and bodies and tending to each person in the relationship with loving care and empathy is necessary for the relationship to thrive.

You Have the Key—Now Unlock Your *Shameless Sex*

By reading this book, you've already embarked on your personal journey toward redefining and re-creating the sex and relationships you desire. As you continue your journey, let the *Shameless Sex* Philosophy guide you. Remember:

Your inner erotic landscape is totally unique and 100 percent normal. As long as you abide by the "all consensual sex is good sex" motto, you have the freedom to explore whatever you fancy. If you think your experiences and desires aren't the "norm," welcome to the club. You're not broken, and it's normal for people to encounter a time in their lives when they feel as though they do not fit in.

Your brain is your largest sex organ, and while certain challenges are physiological, most are related to your personal beliefs and perspectives, based on your programming and what was "given" to you without your consent. The brain is highly malleable, and this provides hope for obtaining the change you are seeking and that you deserve.

Forget everything you were told about how sex and relationships *should* be unless those things are truly an intrinsic part of you, because what you crave sexually matters.

Your sexuality is fluid and exists on a continuum, so it's completely valid if and when that changes. You're always evolving, and sexual pleasure is an important aspect of your transformative process, as it holds the true essence of who you are as an erotic being.

Finally, when in doubt, cultivating presence and self-awareness, strengthening communication and boundary skills, and approaching sexuality with compassion for yourself and any intimate partner you encounter, while continuously sharing your needs, are the best tools to add to your sex and relationship tool kit. In closing, when all else fails, simply press pause, *then go slower than slow and then slower than that.*

We love you. Thank you for being part of the

SHAMELESS SEX REVOLUTION!

Ciao for now . . . Amy & April

Acknowledgments

This book (and our podcast) would never have been possible without the people listed here. We want to honor and acknowledge each and every one of you and shower you with immense gratitude:

SHAMELESS SEX LISTENERS: First and foremost, you inspire us day after day by making this journey perpetually rewarding. Your support through reviews, feedback, and heartfelt testimonials about how we've changed your life gives us the fuel that continues to ignite our shameless fire. Thank you for believing in us—we love you *Shameless Sex* Revolutionaries!

OUR MOMS: Janis Baldwin for trusting the vision and creating Pure Pleasure Shop with your daughter, for listening to every single episode of *Shameless Sex*, and for your tenacity and strength. Barbi for always believing your daughter could change the world and for demonstrating what hard work and dedication look like. Thank you for being powerhouse mothers and incredible women.

OUR FRIENDS: For putting up with us as we went a little cuckoo and became full hermits while writing this book. Your love and support mean the world to us. Thank you for being there. We are so lucky to have you in our lives! You are amazing. Thank you for being our friends.

OUR PARTNERS: For seeing our gifts, encouraging our growth, and loving us as we pour our hearts and souls into this work, knowing how important it is to the world. Thank you for understanding the deep bond of "Chip and Dip" as non-sexual life partners because, as you know, we come as a packaged deal. If it ever feels difficult having a partner who talks openly to hundreds of thousands of people about sex and relation-ships, just remember how much we truly appreciate the way you support us sharing ourselves shamelessly.

THE BENBELLA TEAM: For trusting our mission and helping us see it through, especially Leah Wilson and Leah Baxter (the Leahs) for spend-ing countless hours refining our message—we hope you learned a thing or two during the process and that you had some good laughs too.

OUR LITERARY AGENT: Mark Falkin for sharing your wisdom in the literary world and for sending us an email on a whim asking if we ever considered writing a book. Your auspicious timing helped push us into creating something we had been wanting to do for years.

THE ILLUSTRATORS: Glen Colligan and Stacey Shweeso for taking on a project completely out of your comfort zones, for accommodat-ing every detailed request while creating everything so quickly, and for your humor. Glen, thank you for being the best big bro a sister could ever ask for.

DR. EMILY MORSE: For being a sex podcast pioneer and helping normalize conversations around sex. You inspired us to have a podcast and supported us every step of the way. Thank you for your expertise and friendship. You are the best out there, and we will always love and respect you.

HOT OCTOPUSS AND ÜBERLUBE: For making the best sex toys and lube on the market, for fully backing our creative endeavors with the podcast and the book, and for loving us like family and treating us like royalty. We love you more than you will ever know.

OUR TEACHERS AND MENTORS: Especially all of the educators, therapists, doctors, authors, and other incredible humans who have guested on *Shameless Sex*. Thank you for sharing your knowledge and contributing your expertise. It's a privilege to continue receiving sex education from all of you. You are inspiring more sex positivity and helping to change the world.

OUR FUR BABIES: Legend and Perry for your unconditional love and cuteness, for sitting on our laps while we endlessly sat in front of our laptops, for motivating us to get our asses outside to take screen breaks, for being our children, and for making us laugh all the time. You make life better and our hearts bigger, and we love you even though you'll never read this.

Index

About the Authors

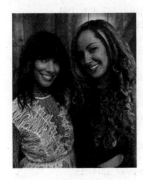

Amy Baldwin (right) is a sex educator and sex and relationship coach trained in both the Somatica and Hakomi Methods. Amy is also the lead educator for überlube, co-owner of a mother-daughter owned online pleasure boutique called Pure Pleasure Shop, and was voted Sexpert of the Year within the pleasure products industry.

April Lampert (left) is co-owner and chief sales and partnerships officer of Hot Octopuss, an innovative and award-winning sex toy company. She was voted Woman of the Year in the pleasure products industry and has been educating people about sexual pleasure and sex toys at a global scale since 2008.

Together, Amy and April created the *Shameless Sex* podcast, inspiring radical self-love, sexual empowerment, and shame-free intimacy. *Shameless Sex* is known for its unabashed real talk about sexuality with a playful twist, and has been featured in mainstream media outlets such as

Cosmopolitan, Women's Health, Men's Health, Huffington Post, GQ, and *Maxim*, among other platforms.

shamelesssex.com

@ShamelessSexPodcast

@ShamelessSexPodcast

@ShamelessSexPodcast